THE
6 KEYS

Also by Jillian Michaels

Winning by Losing: Drop the Weight, Change Your Life

Making the Cut: The 30-Day Diet and Fitness Plan for the Strongest, Sexiest You

Master Your Metabolism: The 3 Diet Secrets to Naturally Balancing Your Hormones for a Hot and Healthy Body!

The Master Your Metabolism Calorie Counter

The Master Your Metabolism Cookbook

Unlimited: How to Build an Exceptional Life

Slim for Life: My Insider Secrets to Simple, Fast, and Lasting Weight Loss

Yeah Baby! The Modern Mama's Guide to Mastering Pregnancy, Having a Healthy Baby, and Bouncing Back Better Than Ever

THE

6KEYS

Unlock Your Genetic Potential for
Ageless Strength, Health, and Beauty

JILLIAN MICHAELS
with Myatt Murphy

LITTLE, BROWN SPARK
New York Boston London

Copyright © 2018 by Jillian Michaels

Hachette Book Group supports the right to free expression and the value of copyright. The purpose of copyright is to encourage writers and artists to produce the creative works that enrich our culture.

The scanning, uploading, and distribution of this book without permission is a theft of the author's intellectual property. If you would like permission to use material from the book (other than for review purposes), please contact permissions@hbgusa.com. Thank you for your support of the author's rights.

Little, Brown Spark
Hachette Book Group
1290 Avenue of the Americas, New York, NY 10104
littlebrownspark.com

Originally published in hardcover by Little, Brown Spark, December 2018
First Little, Brown Spark paperback edition, December 2020

Little, Brown Spark is an imprint of Little, Brown and Company, a division of Hachette Book Group, Inc. The Little, Brown Spark name and logo are trademarks of Hachette Book Group, Inc.

The publisher is not responsible for websites (or their content) that are not owned by the publisher.

The Hachette Speakers Bureau provides a wide range of authors for speaking events. To find out more, go to hachettespeakersbureau.com or call (866) 376-6591.

ISBN 978-0-316-44864-2 (hc) / 978-0-316-44863-5 (pb)
LCCN 2018952826

Printing 1, 2020

LSC-C

Printed in the United States of America

This one is for my little girl, Lukensia Michaels-Rhoades.

You will always be my baby, but watching you grow into an incredible and beautiful young woman inside and out has been one of the greatest highlights of my life.
While this book is for men and women alike, as a woman, you will face particular prejudices and judgments as you age that men might not. Never believe the haters or the naysayers. When they try to tell you what you can or can't do, remember that's a projection of their limitations, not yours.
With every passing day you become wiser, smarter, stronger, and even more beautiful. The world is your oyster, the future is bright, and life is what you make it. Make it beautiful, angel. You deserve it. Fill your heart with empathy, your mind with hope, and your body with vigor. Unleash yourself on the world and live your truest, most passionate, adventurous life!

Contents

THE
6 KEYS

Introduction

We've all heard that old saying that nothing in life is certain but death and taxes. The taxes I can't help you with, but did you know there is nothing in our genes that tells us to die?

That's right—NOTHING.

So, the big question is: why aren't we immortal? Why does one person barely make it to retirement age while another gets to blow out candles on their ninety-eighth birthday? Why are some more susceptible to certain health issues as they get older (like Alzheimer's, cancer, and heart disease), while others seem immune? Why do some people look frail, gray, and shriveled as they age, while others remain vigorous, potent, and powerful?

If you haven't asked these questions yet, at some point in your life, you will.

The need to truly understand everything about growing older hit me on a random night out at a local Santa Monica beer garden with my younger siblings. Much younger, in fact—my brother is twenty-eight and my little sister is just twenty-four. Admittedly, I don't find myself at bars filled with millennials often, but my brother had recently had his heart crushed in a breakup and my sister and I were determined to help him get over it.

So there I was, forty-three years old, hanging out at a bar

packed with twenty-somethings, dressed low-key: no makeup, hair in a ball cap, wearing a pair of jeans, a T-shirt, and sneakers.

And I get carded—for real.

At first, I was like, this guy either thinks I'm some sort of undercover cop or he feels bad for me. But no. He took my ID, glanced at it, looked back up, immediately did a double-take and said, "Wow! You've maintained really well."

My little sister—the highly educated, idealistic, politically correct young woman that she is—was furious and offended on my behalf. I, on the other hand, was ecstatic. I thanked him and could tell he was genuinely shocked to discover I was forty-three years old, but as I walked away, something struck me.

Why was he so shocked?

In my mind, I looked and felt my age: I felt wiser, stronger, and more successful than when I was younger, possessing a confidence that only comes with time and experience. So why wasn't *that* what forty-something looked like to him?

As the night went on and I mingled among the crowd, people continued to be astonished by my age.

"You do NOT look forty-three!"

"You don't SEEM like you're forty-three!"

At first, I was super flattered. But by the eighth person, I started to get annoyed. *What the hell?* I thought. *What exactly is forty-three supposed to be and look like anyway? Why does everyone else think forty-three is old?* More important, what do *you* believe forty-plus is supposed to look and feel like?

Let me guess. Getting older means you're most likely going to be:

- Tired (well, I can feel a little tired, but I blame that one on my kids—not my biology)

- Forgetful and out of touch
- Overweight and out of shape
- Inflexible and achy all the time
- Experiencing hair loss and gray hair
- Dealing with sagging, wrinkled skin
- Heading into pre-menopause or menopause
- Having trouble getting or keeping an erection (not for me of course, but this one's for you, my male readers)

Well, guess what? I am none of the above.

In fact, I am the exact opposite of all of the above. (Okay, to be honest, I am super forgetful, but that's nothing new. I was born with that one.)

For weeks after that night out with my siblings, I paid attention to everyone around me and tried to guess people's ages in my head. I couldn't help wondering how people of the same age could be so different from one another when it came to their energy level, immunity, memory, productivity, functionality, personality, and physical appearance. I couldn't stop thinking about the causes for this huge variance in how people age. I knew I needed to explore, dissect, and decode the habits and behaviors of those who seem to defy aging. My fascination with aging led to the book you now hold in your hands.

The 6 Keys is the most comprehensive and effective approach to anti-aging on the market. And while I know that term has become a dirty word in most PC circles, can we just call a spade a spade? This book isn't about being afraid to get older—it's about aging well!

It reveals everything we presently know (not just bits and pieces) about how we age and integrates all that information into one approach that optimizes our genetics and exploits our physiological potential. It's not a book full of false promises and magic-bullet solutions based on what's trending. Instead, it's literally an owner's manual for a long-lived body, complete with honest instruction. It's science, not fiction. And while it's true that results may vary based on your dedication, the information herein is irrefutable and extremely potent when applied.

Now, maybe you don't really care about all that science stuff and it seems overwhelming. And yes, even though this book is about a lot more than looks, let's level with each other: maybe you just want to know how to look hot at fifty, sixty, and beyond. If that's the case, not to worry. In fact, good for you!

There is nothing wrong with caring about your appearance, provided you don't allow it to define your self-worth. And if you've picked up this book because that's what you care about, that's perfectly okay. Because if you're looking for a fountain of youth, this book will be as close as you can get.

Aging gracefully doesn't have to mean giving up and accepting decay. It means keeping yourself in fantastic health, inside and out, for a hell of a long time. After all, would you want to live in a dilapidated home? Should you neglect your car until it breaks down? Would you wear stained, dirty, or wrinkled clothes (unless you're in the privacy of your home on a Netflix binge)? Of course not. There's a sense of pride and self-worth that comes along with caring about yourself—and for yourself. This is your body we are talking about—your one and only true home. You know, that physical shell that quite literally *houses* you for your entire life. And it's the only one you're ever going to get, so you should care for it and about it! How it looks. How it feels. How it performs. And, most important, how long it lasts.

So just in case you mistakenly feel that caring about your appearance, sex life, energy, and vigor is arrogant, selfish, or shallow, this book will put that notion to bed for good. How you feel about yourself, carry yourself, and present yourself dramatically impacts the way you relate to your environment and other people in it, which in turn dramatically impacts your quality of life and how you age. I mean, longevity is great, but longevity without vitality, immunity, and everything else I've mentioned— well, that's not so great. But you *can* have it all. This book will teach you how.

Want in? Read on.

Part 1

THE LOCK

Before you can unlock aging, you need to understand the mistaken beliefs most of us have about the aging process.

There are so many misconceptions about what's really bolting that door shut and keeping us from aging on our own terms. Is it genetics? Is it too much sun? Is it every bad habit you ever had in your life coming back to haunt you? The fact is, that lock is a culmination of a lot of things. But it's knowing which ones are the most important to focus on that makes the lock much easier to open.

We'll begin by looking at the different ways we define our age, and how all of those various ways come together to make us feel or appear our true age. I'll then explain the facts around what aging really is and what others believe about why we have to grow old in the first place. I mean, there has to be a valid reason, right? Finally, I will share with you how I came to discover the 6 Keys among the emerging science that is now transforming how researchers and scientists perceive and address aging.

CHAPTER 1

Which Age Defines You?

I have a question for you: how do *you* want to age?

- Do you want to live to 150—or even 200? Professor Stuart Kim of Stanford University believes the first person to do so is alive right now!
- Would you like to be able to reprogram your body—and the bodies of your children—to make it impossible for cancer to grow as you get older? Sounds impossible, but we're a lot closer to doing that than you might think.
- Would you like to be in amazing shape—possibly the best shape of your life—at fifty, sixty, seventy, eighty, or even ninety? Yuichiro Miura scaled Everest at eighty, Jack Nicklaus shot a hole in one at seventy-five, and Diana Nyad swam 110 miles from Cuba to Florida when she was sixty-four. One of the world's most lauded yoga instructors, Tao Porchon-Lynch, is one hundred. And at fifty-four, Texas native Mark Jordan set a Guinness World Record in 2015 for the most pull-ups in a twenty-four-hour period (4,321!).

I know what you're thinking. I've picked genetic anomalies, wealthy elites, or lifelong athletes—all outliers of epic proportion, right?

Wrong.

It's *never* too late, and the things you think are impossible or out of your reach aren't—not by a long shot. For the first time in human history, thanks to advancements in medical science, we have made incredible discoveries that help us understand not only why and how we age but how to slow and even reverse aging and avoid age-related illness.

There are keys—six to be exact—that collectively open that door, and ways to make those 6 Keys turn, without fail, in the right direction.

Now, these accomplishments aren't effortless. They require dedication, appreciation, and a profound love for yourself. They require a strong understanding of the science of aging, immunity, longevity, and vitality. They require the courage to make necessary changes—at any age. And perhaps most important, they require an open mind, a shift in thinking, and a new perspective about aging.

But before we dig in to the 6 Keys, just between us, tell me: how old are you? I mean, really.

Sorry, too personal of a question? Okay, I get it, but the whole point here is that it's nothing to be ashamed of. And in fact, redefining age in your mind will be a pretty critical component to how you age. So, tell me.

In truth, I don't care about this number. I am actually asking to illustrate a point. Your "age" has many different factors that you are likely not considering, and each dramatically impacts the others to cumulatively affect how you look, feel, and perform over time.

- For starters, there's your **chronological** age, which is the number dictated by your birth certificate. It's officially how long you've been alive and technically the age you can't escape. Not to worry. Spend some time with me and you won't want to escape.

- There's your **biological** (or **physiological**) age, which is how old your body "seems" based on how well you move, look, and function. It's an age that can vary depending on a number of factors, such as lifestyle choices, diet, genetics, stress, and bad habits.

- There's your **emotional** age, which is how well you manage your feelings. For example, do you handle stressful situations more rationally than someone your chronological age, or instead tend to act like a hot mess?

- There's your **social** age, which is based on the expectations society imposes on us about when life's major moments should occur (such as graduating from high school, starting a family, or retiring), and about what appropriate or inappropriate behavior should be for someone of a particular age.

- Finally, there's your **psychological** age, better known as "how old do you feel?" It's the age that's entirely up to you because it's however you see and carry yourself. That can mean being the young-at-heart type or considering yourself an old soul—that sort of thing.

HOW ALL OF YOUR AGES ADD UP

If you've been trying to cheat time by focusing strictly on your biological age (through exercise, diet, supplements, creams, etc.), I commend your efforts, but it's utterly incomplete. The first step in turning that around is understanding that all of your ages—including your emotional, social, and psychological ages—must be considered as a whole in order for your actions to be effective.

For example, you may not think that acting irrationally would age you faster—but it could. Many studies have shown that the higher your emotional intelligence—your ability to recognize and understand emotions in yourself (and others) and to use this awareness to manage your behavior and relationships—the more likely you are to make better decisions, manage anxiety,[1] and be more resilient to stress,[2] all of which can help you age well.

The same respect should be paid to your social age. Society pretty much dictates exactly when we should be hitting various milestones in our lives. In your late teens, you graduate high school, and by your early twenties, you better be at the start of your career. Between your late twenties and early thirties, you settle down and start building a family. By your forties, if you change careers or do something profoundly stupid, no one bats an eye—you get a free pass because you're officially in a midlife crisis. Hit your mid-sixties and it's time to retire. And that's pretty much the social age rat race in a nutshell.

Nail these markers at the expected times and your social age is right on track. But if you dare deviate, your social age may fall much younger or older than the norm, which could affect you in ways you might not expect. Being a teenage mom, feeling the pressure to be in a serious relationship or on a career track, going back to school in your thirties, or not being financially able to retire are just a few deviations from the norm that could bring on what scientists call "social stress."

Research[3] has shown that social stress may actually interfere with cellular aging and DNA repair, and according to recent data,[4] where you rank within the social hierarchy could play a major role in how vulnerable you are to chronic stress. Struggling in social settings may also put you at a greater risk for mental and physical health problems,[5] particularly depression and anxiety—two conditions that make you more vulnerable to accelerated aging[6] for many reasons, such as lowering your testosterone levels[7] and impairing white blood cells[8] (the cells that protect your body from diseases and infections).

Finally, there's the often disregarded but equally important psychological age. Age can be a self-fulfilling prophecy. What you believe affects your behavior, and how you behave affects your reality. If you believe you're frail and tired, you'll stop moving your body in ways that help with bone density, flexibility, mobility, etc.—so you'll literally become frail and tired. If you feel ineffectual or "outdated," you'll stop using your mind in ways that keep it sharp. Simply put: once you accept you're old— you become old.

Your psychological age affects your body *and* your mind. New research[9] from North Carolina State University found that having a positive attitude about aging makes older adults more resilient under stress, while a different study found that having a negative attitude was confirmed[10] to affect physical and cognitive health in later years. To make matters worse, research[11] led by the Yale School of Public Health discovered that people with negative beliefs about aging are also more likely to have brain changes associated with Alzheimer's disease. Simply believing that getting older sucks creates stress that can cause pathological brain changes!

Why do I bring all of this up? Because what you're about to embark upon with the 6 Keys goes beyond the conventional approach typically explored in most anti-aging programs. You'll go beyond improving your biological age, because in order to truly change our bodies, we first need to change our minds: the way we think, the things we believe, and subsequently the way we behave. Accepting this reality is the first step.

It is possible to decide how you age. You can have a long, tremendous, spectacular, healthy life—but not without giving yourself over to the aging process mentally and physically. You will need faith. Faith in the science, faith in the strategy, but most important, faith in your ability to believe it and achieve it.

And I'll tell you this much: if I can do it, you can do it. There is nothing exceptional about me. Don't get me wrong, I feel capable and worthy of all things great that life has to offer, but I know you are, too. I'm not beautiful like a supermodel, I'm not a genius, I wasn't born into money, and I have zero special skills or talents.

Now, what I do have working for me is that I had great teachers. Teachers who believed in me when I didn't believe in myself. Teachers who showed me that I was capable and who gave me the tools and proper information so that when I took action, I got powerful results that helped reinforce my belief in the process, my abilities, and my motivation. And that's what I'm going to do for you with the 6 Keys.

You picked up this book, so you must believe that I know what I'm doing. You've likely seen the results I've helped people achieve over the years, and hopefully, you're looking at me and thinking that I am doing pretty well at forty-four. So, if you believe in me, know that I believe in you, and by this virtuous circle, you ultimately must believe in yourself.

And maybe you think that's bullsh*t. I've never met you, so how can I possibly believe in you? I know it because I know the science. I know that when applied, the results are inevitable. Beyond the hundreds of studies I've read, many of which I'll discuss—I'm living proof. Knowledge is power. It empowers us to make informed decisions and take precise, deliberate actions that yield incredible results.

Yes, it is possible to look your best, feel your best, fend off disease, stay sharp, and be your most robust, fit, and flourishing self for years to come. And soon, you'll have the keys to making that possibility a reality.

All that said, as mentioned, I make no false promises and offer no magic bullets. These changes will require some work, vulnerability, and sacrifice. Anything worth having always does. And in order to follow through on all those things, you need to have a *why*. I'm sure you've heard me toss this quote out a thousand times, and for good reason: "If you have a *why* to live for... you can tolerate any *how*." The *how* being the work associated with achieving the goal.

So, I need you to think deeply about *why* this matters to you. How will your life be positively impacted by the changes you are about to make? And I don't mean sweeping generalizations like "I'll look better" or "I'll feel better." I mean specifics to which you can form an emotional attachment.

I already know why aging badly isn't on my agenda. Because I love being on the slopes with my kids, not waiting for them at the bottom of the mountain with hot chocolate.

I love being strong physically because I find it empowers me in all facets of my life and reminds me of my resilience and ability to endure, persevere, and overcome adversity.

I love that professionally I have only continued to grow more successful as I've gotten older because I don't just talk my message—I live it.

I love feeling good about how I have "maintained," because it gives me confidence in all my interactions.

I love that at forty-four, I am far more fit than I was at

thirty-four — or even twenty-four. Because it fills me with hope and positivity for what is yet to come.

I love that I am super comfortable in a two-piece.

I love that I am doing everything in my power to fend off cancer, Alzheimer's, and heart disease. And even if they do get me, I will have zero regrets around how I tried to avoid it.

I could go on and on and on here . . . but that is a book unto itself, and this book is about you. So, I'll stop, as I'm sure you get the idea.

The bottom line is that I know age doesn't have to be a slow descent into decrepitude. It is possible to age fully empowered with grace, beauty, wisdom, and integrity. I have defied and will continue to defy preconceived notions about aging. I will redefine it on my own terms — physically and psychologically.

So the real question is: how 'bout you?

CHAPTER 2

The Truth About Aging

What *is* aging anyway? Think you know? Think again.

Aging is one of the most complex biological processes in existence, and defining it is not easy—even for the experts. I've heard scientists call aging "the time-based breakdown of the physiological functions needed to survive and reproduce." I've heard other experts refer to it as "the accumulation of changes in a human being over time encompassing physical, psychological, and social changes."

But in the most general terms, aging is just the process of growing older—period.

It's a process that affects almost all of the body's systems and the cells of every major organ at rates that can vary greatly from person to person. How well we age is typically defined by changes in our appearance, reaction times, metabolism, memory functions, fitness levels, sex drive, and the ability to see, hear, and even smell. Other signs of aging are a decrease in organ function, a weaker immune system, and various hormonal changes, just to name a few.

But a better way to look at it may be to understand what aging is *not*.

Aging is not the enemy

Aging is a natural and normal process. It can make us wiser, smarter, and stronger—both physically and emotionally. I'm proud of my age. Literally. Proud of it. Because it *is* an accomplishment. Life is not about perfection. It's about progress. And progress only comes with age. I have survived forty-four years on this planet. In that time, I have done some great things and some stupid things—but each of them has helped me grow and made me who I am today. I truly believe that ubiquitous quotation: "The only person you should try to be better than is the person you were yesterday." And I am, with every passing day.

I once trained a sixty-five-year-old woman and her thirty-year-old daughter. The sixty-five-year-old was stronger—by far. She could do eighty-pound lat pull-downs—the daughter could only handle sixty-five pounds. She could leg-press two hundred pounds! Her daughter could only do a hundred and forty. And the list goes on.

It was fascinating. I figured the disparity couldn't be caused by genes, because the daughter had her mom's genes. It wasn't that the mom was a lifelong athlete—she wasn't. That said, she had survived a hell of a lot in her life, and I came to the conclusion that her mental resilience and psychological fortitude had transformed into a manifestation of physical strength. This woman had walked through fire, survived it, and felt anything else was child's play. So a two-hundred-pound leg press? Please—easy!

Aging is not "time"

The passing of time is not the primary cause of decrepitude! The choices we make regarding the way we live are what cause our bodies to decay quickly or maintain and thrive.

Ultimately, we are not immortal, and eventually, we will die. But if you make the right choices, you will get many more years and extremely vigorous ones at that.

Aging isn't what kills you

That's right! Aging isn't the reason we actually die. Research[1] has shown that the very notion that people die of "old age" is a complete fallacy.

It is true that as we get older, some age-related changes have a greater impact than others. But while these changes may make us more susceptible to disease, they don't inevitably lead to age-related pathologies such as type-2 diabetes, hypertension, heart disease, or dementia.

WHY DO WE AGE?

Much like the science of nutrition and metabolism, the science of aging has been convoluted. There have been many theories and very little science up until relatively recently.

For centuries, philosophers and researchers have debated the true causes of aging. In fact, in 1990, Russian biologist and aging expert Zhores Medvedev categorized[2] more than three hundred different theories of aging. That's not a typo—I said three hundred different theories! (Side note: as I write this, Medvedev is ninety-two years old and still kicking, so maybe the secret to defying aging is simply researching it—why do you think I wrote this book? Just sayin'. But I digress.)

Now, while there have been many theories over the years on this topic, there are only a couple that have truly endured.

Some say it's damage

Some theories propose that aging is the result of a constant assault on various molecules and cells in our bodies, ranging from proteins to DNA. Everything from exposure to the environment and toxic by-products (such as unstable atoms, ions, or molecules known as free radicals) to inefficiencies in our body's natural repair systems causes this damage, according to the theories. The damage accumulates like junk inside us throughout our entire lifespan, prompting some biological systems to fail, which in turn causes and accelerates the aging process. In fact, almost all research and observation points to this being true. And while it isn't quite that simple — our bodies react to these stressors differently based on our genetics — it's without doubt a major component.

However, aging isn't all about wear and tear. Your body isn't like some old jalopy that's broken down and busted. Or is it? Let's think about this for a second. If we did use this analogy, what if that car had been cared for and maintained with routine service? What if it were kept garaged, given high-quality fuel, the spark plugs and oil changed regularly, and so on? That car would do a hell of a lot better and be around a hell of a lot longer than if it hadn't been well maintained.

Sure, our bodies take a beating as we speed through life, but in many cases, that damage can be managed, prevented, and in some cases even reversed with the proper nutrition, stress management, lifestyle, and so on. Our bodies have the ability to repair, regenerate, or replace most of our cells and molecules. So, aging may be in small part due to wear and tear, but it's in large part due to neglect.

Phew. That was a long walk to get a sandwich, but you get it now, right?

The good news is that much of the damage can be fixed or, better yet, prevented from happening in the first place — once you understand the 6 Keys.

Some say it's destiny

There are some that theorize aging is predetermined, that it is encoded into our genes and occurs on a fixed schedule triggered by those genes.

Imagine there's some sort of preordained blueprint that runs its course, then causes certain genetically regulated processes to take over and signal, "Okay, it's time for you to go now!" It's as if there's a kind of molecular clock (or series of clocks) that activates a sequence of age-related changes and diseases.

Here are two examples of "destiny" theories:

• In 1952, biologist Sir Peter Medawar theorized that we age so that the risk of passing on the harmful mutations that tend to spring up in our genes after reproduction don't get passed on to future generations. Meaning: the older we get, the more mutations we tend to rack up, so to prevent those mutations from affecting our progeny — our bodies start to die to keep us from having kids.

• In 1977, biologist Thomas Kirkwood proposed that we only have a limited amount of energy, which is divided between reproductive activities and everything else that keeps our bodies functioning. Once we use up that energy, it takes away from the body's perfectly balanced ability to maintain itself, allowing mutations and other cellular damage to occur over time.

Ultimately, the destiny theories are predominantly rooted in the fact that we wear out our usefulness. But the question is… when? At forty, ninety, two hundred?

Obviously we already know that this answer can vary tremendously from person to person, and *that* is where the 6 Keys come in to play. There is no true evidence of a genetic time bomb that says "decay." If there were, then aging and dying would happen at the same time for everyone. For example: all Pacific salmon breed, then die soon afterward. Human beings don't function that way.

I have met plenty of people who had no children and died early. I have also met plenty of people who have had many kids and lived well into their nineties or even became centenarians. My great-grandmother was one of them—she had six kids! And the fact that many people live well into their nineties proves the destiny theory is at best terribly incomplete and at worst total bull.

There is lots of evidence that suggests aging is triggered by a host of variables (many quite manageable). So if I don't subscribe to destiny theories, then why even mention them? Several reasons.

First, to cover my ass. People will criticize this book because it harms their agenda. Selling sickness is a business, and many associate age with sickness. I mean, look at what the drug companies did with menopause, for God's sake. They turned a perfectly normal biological process that's been happening since the existence of our species into a disease that needs to be medicated. The great irony here is that many studies show it's the synthetic hormones and drugs people take to control menopause that actually accelerate disease.

Second, if you're vulnerable to destiny theory, it's imperative we bring it up and refute it because we know for a fact that what we believe affects how we behave—and how we behave dictates our reality. So if you think you're aging poorly, you act like you're aging poorly, and you start becoming less active, etc. It becomes a self-fulfilling prophecy.

Now, before we move on, there is one component of destiny theory that is legit—sorta. It's that the interactions between the nervous and endocrine systems (neuroendocrinology) dictate many aspects of the aging process and could trigger that genetic time bomb I crapped all over earlier. But, and this is a big *but,* what is messing up our neuroendocrinology? And this is where the nuance comes in. It would seem that accumulative damage could screw that up.

There are plenty of damage-buildup theories that acknowledge that genes and hormones have a hand in aging. Conversely, many destiny theories tip their hat to the fact that internal and external damage could impact aging to an extent. That's why some believe—and I'm one of them—that the smartest way to approach aging is to acknowledge that it is a combination of separate underlying processes collectively undermining many of our body's systems simultaneously.

In other words, the answers lie in the processes of aging and what we can do to tip the scales in our favor.

CHAPTER 3

The 6 Keys to Unlock Longevity and Vitality

When I first began looking for the keys to aging, I didn't need to go very far, since I had already found one when researching my bestselling book *Master Your Metabolism*.

Back then, I looked at metabolism strictly from a weight-loss and overall health perspective, teaching readers how to bring their out-of-whack hormones back in sync. But along the way, my fascination with how our metabolism works kept steering me toward the connection between metabolism and aging. As it turns out, the very act of metabolizing food stresses our bodies in a way that could accelerate the aging process. In other words, the more you eat, the more effort your body spends extracting energy from food. All that effort might age you faster than you would like.

I also came to discover that when you restrict calories, there's an almost linear increase in life span—so the less you eat, the longer you live. The anti-aging merit of calorie restriction (a reduction in caloric intake while consuming sufficient quantities of vitamins, minerals, and other essential nutrients) has been proven to extend life span across a variety of species, not just our own—from roundworms to rats and, most recently, rhesus monkeys. Researchers at the University of Wisconsin–Madison and the National Institute on Aging discovered[1] that a rhesus monkey placed on a 30 percent calorie restriction diet could live up to forty-three years (the equivalent of 130 human years), breaking longevity records for the species.

How does science explain it? Is it because metabolizing fewer calories results in less stress on the body? Could the absence of key nutrients be triggering defense mechanisms that shield the body from health issues? Is it because calorie restriction (at least in overweight subjects) enhances the function of mitochondria, the little organelles inside your cells that produce 90 percent of the energy required to keep you alive? I quickly found out that nothing is being discounted when it comes to metabolism's role in aging. But it's important to note that metabolism is not the only player at work here.

The deeper I dove into the research, the more I gravitated toward the emerging field of *geroscience,* which looks at the relationship between aging and disease, or in other words, how to slow aging and stay super healthy for a really long time.

Scientists are now pursuing a more thorough understanding of the mechanisms of aging, one that can answer questions about the biological processes responsible for a decrease in bone and muscle strength, higher vulnerability to disease, impaired overall function, and all the other consequences of aging we're less than happy about. The only issue is that they're not all on the same page just yet when it comes to which processes of aging to target.

THE CONSENSUS OF 6 KEYS

Many geroscientists point to a pioneering paper[2] published in 2013 that proposed there are nine causes, or hallmarks, of aging. Other leading scientists are more interested in the effects, or pillars, of certain processes that change as we age.[3] What I've done in this book is analyze both the hallmarks *and* the pillars together in order to give you the smartest strategy that provides the most comprehensive and effective approach to unlocking your healthiest, strongest self.

Ultimately, no single factor is truly independent from — or more important than — the rest, and it's the intertwining of these causes and effects that ultimately ages us. So while some researchers are busy seeking precise ways to cure age-related issues and diseases like hypertension, cancer, and Alzheimer's individually, others are taking a broader viewpoint. They are more interested in pinpointing the influences on how we age so that by targeting "key" areas they can potentially delay and diminish every age-related issue all at once. That's what the 6 Keys is all about. I've found those "key" areas that decide how we age from head to toe — inside and out.

Just as metabolism is a factor in many contemporary theories of aging, there are a few other common threads that always pop up. In fact there are six essential cellular and molecular areas and/or processes that are consistently linked to aging. It's these 6 Keys that are the biggest power players in making or breaking how well we age.

The First Key is mastering your macromolecules: As we get older, macromolecules can either become damaged (DNA, lipids, and proteins) or accumulate (free radicals and damaged proteins). This can cause specific age-related issues and diseases, such as wrinkles, gray hair, organ failure, and even Alzheimer's. The First Key is to take every possible step to minimize detrimental changes to our macromolecules.

The Second Key is engineering your epigenetics: Our environment—which can include pollutants, bad habits, medications, and diet—and even how our ancestors lived can affect how our genes work and influence our development, health, and how fast or slowly we age. The Second Key is to control variable factors that can affect your genes—for better or for worse.

The Third Key is strong-arming your stress: Researchers now know there's a common thread among animals that live the longest: their cells are more resistant to a variety of stressors. People that live longer tend to recover faster from the physical wear and tear of activity, bounce back better from psychological trauma, and suffer less damage from stress-related hormones such as cortisol and adrenaline. The Third Key is about becoming more resilient to stress, along with reducing stress at every level, especially the stress that you can't see and have no idea exists in the first place.

The Fourth Key is owning your inflammation: There is a slow, gradual increase in inflammation within the body as we age, and low-level chronic inflammation is destructive—a phenomenon known as "inflamm-*aging*." There are a host of internal and external factors that can cause it, from what we throw in our bellies as food to the bacteria that actually live there. The Fourth Key is all about preventing chronic, unhealthy inflammation.

The Fifth Key is managing your metabolism: Oh, but you should have seen that one coming, right? The thing is, beyond what I've already shared with you about how metabolizing food causes stress that may age us, there is even more to unravel regarding our metabolism's role in either reversing or revving up aging. The Fifth Key requires us to look at the many ways you can either manipulate or harness the power of your metabolism to work for you.

The Sixth Key is tackling your telomeres: Telomeres are the protective tips at the end of each DNA strand. They shorten as we age, but this doesn't have to be inevitable. What you eat, how you exercise, and even how anxious or depressed you feel can play a part in keeping your telomeres long and strong. The Sixth Key lies in delaying the fraying of your telomeres.

So there you have it. The 6 Keys—ta da! For real, though, understanding and manipulating these six factors will literally change your life. Most books, papers, studies, and programs focus on one of the six. There are a handful of programs that have touched on two of these age inciters—usually metabolism and inflammation. But until now, no one has ever constructed a solution that addresses all six simultaneously. Literally no one has ever conceived a multi-level strategy that is based on *all* of the latest cutting-edge science on aging and targets *all* the culprits with one unified strategy.

In large part, this is because doctors and scientists subspecialize—they work in their field and stay in their lane. They focus on the micro, not the macro. And in all fairness, the only way to truly understand something is to do a deep and focused dive into it. However, at some point, someone has to bring all the pieces together in order to effectively determine a 360-degree solution. It's one big 3-D puzzle, and if one piece is missing, the solution is incomplete.

All six age inciters must be addressed simultaneously so that you can beat age-related diseases and become the healthiest, sexiest, most vital, energized version of yourself for decades to come. You need a truly comprehensive and cohesive strategy to optimize your genetic potential and gain the greatest possible control over how you age.

That is exactly what the 6 Keys is all about.

The 6 Keys is a journey into the realm of superhumanity, one rooted in science as opposed to magic and myth. It reveals the absolute principles underlying longevity and vitality, offering a way of life that restores, protects, and optimizes human performance, immunity, potency, and vigor. This is not a traditional program or plan, and it's not a fad or trend—it's a way to harness the life force incarnate.

In the chapters to come, you'll learn everything there is to know about all six age inciters and how to address each one through a streamlined action strategy that delivers desired results. And when I say desired, I mean like really f'ing amazing results. So if you're ready for me to turn the keys over to you, here they are. Let's pop this lock and turn back your clock once and for all.

Part 2

THE KEYS

So, you're buckled up and ready for blast off. Fantastic. Real quick, let me lay out for you the journey we'll be taking in order to eliminate any confusion along the way and make this ride as smooth as possible. I want you to understand what you're reading and why, and what to expect when.

We'll start with a deep dive into each of the 6 Keys. Each chapter will first explain what the key is and how it works in your body. Then I'll cover how and why it can incite aging or reverse it. We'll glimpse the future and explore what our current medical researchers are banging away at to make immortality inevitable (kidding—sorta). And most important, we'll wrap each chapter with what we know *now* to make the key work for as opposed to against us.

This is where I'll introduce the broad strokes of anti-aging and rejuvenation, but we won't dig in to the details until part 3. The reason for this is twofold: first, as you read, you will begin to notice a few themes emerging. Often, an element that impacts one key will also impact several others. In order to avoid redundancy, all the answers will live together in one comprehensive chapter. Second, I don't want to piecemeal the program. There is a lot to take in over the next one hundred or so pages, and in my experience it's far better to set the stage by introducing the key players, inspiring with information, and then empowering with an action and strategy. In part 3 I will tell you exactly how to put all the knowledge and information you'll have just digested to use. And, I've even built a meal plan and fitness regimen into the Jillian Michaels My Fitness App to make this as simple, affordable, and accessible as possible for you. Here is the link to check it out: https://www.jillianmichaels.com/6keys2app.

One caveat before we begin: in some cases, the subject matter can be intense, the information dense, and the verbiage overwhelming. I've done my best to make it as digestible as possible, but should you find yourself checking out at any point, just jump ahead to the plan and implement it. Yes, I would love for you to know the why behind this mind, body, and soul overhaul, but ultimately, it's my job to give you the tools to be successful. And that's what you'll find in part 3. So, as we are about to start with the First Key, remember, you don't need to be a biochemist to get through this. The bottom line will be simple, straightforward, accessible, affordable, and powerful enough to keep you motivated for the rest of your life.

CHAPTER 4

The First Key: Mastering Macromolecules

About 96 percent of your body is a mix of just four separate elements: carbon, hydrogen, oxygen, and nitrogen. But if you need a more impressive number, your body breaks down into more than thirty-seven trillion cells—that's according to researchers who had incredible patience and obviously plenty of time on their hands.

Those cells are your building blocks, and each one serves a purpose. Inside every one of those little suckers are different kinds of molecules that are absolutely essential to how well that cell functions. Four classes of molecules—or macromolecules— are particularly important. You'll recognize three of the four because you eat them every day. They are proteins, carbohydrates, and lipids (fats).

Proteins are a big deal because they not only take up the most room in your cells, but also essentially control everything. You may already know that protein plays a part in building and maintaining muscle, but it also does the same for your bones, blood, organs, and other tissues. Proteins also come in various forms— from enzymes to antibodies—and handle everything from fighting off pathogens to pulling off almost every chemical reaction that happens inside your cells.

Carbohydrates aren't slackers either. They're famous for storing energy in the form of simple sugars for short-term fuel. But carbs also facilitate essential bodily processes like communication among cells and molecules. Carbs are attached to the outside of a cell and act as receptors. So when a cell comes in contact with another cell, the carbs on each cell sense and recognize each other. Carbs create structure within a cell to provide support or offer protection. They also help create a layer around the cell called the glycocalyx, which offers additional protection around the cell membrane. So yeah, carbohydrates play a pretty significant role.

Your lipids (which include fat-soluble vitamins, sterols, waxes, and fats) also store energy. But they have other important jobs like maintaining the structure of your cells' membranes and stabilizing your metabolism and hormone levels.

Surprised that every cell in your body is made up of the three things people have been arguing about whether or not to eat over the last fifty years? Fat-free, no carb, etc. It's all bull. Remember this info the next time a fad diet is repackaged and hawked to you. Your diet should include protein, carbs, and fat. Period. The ratio can vary a bit, but ultimately it's about feeding your cells because you are technically one big mass of all three. And no, this is not a license to eat crap food. It's about quality versions of all three macronutrients, and if you are confused about what exactly that means I will break it down for you in chapter 13. But it's really all just common sense. Eat whole grains, not processed, bleached white flour that's been stripped of its fiber and nutrients. Eat an apple, not processed apple juice that's loaded with high fructose corn syrup and stripped of its fiber, too. Eat wild salmon instead of lunch meat that's heavily processed with chemicals. You get the idea.

The last macromolecule to discuss, nucleic acid, likely will be found on your menu tonight. Nucleic acids are in almost every type of food, but most predominantly in fish (or any form of protein), high-fiber fruit, omega-3 fatty acids, beans, etc. As you digest your food, the nucleic acids inside your food get broken down into nucleotides, which are the molecules that stick together to form your DNA. Literally *all* of your DNA is structured from billions of nucleotide bases.

These molecules—which include ribonucleic acid (RNA), tRNA (transfer RNA), mRNA (messenger RNA), as well as deoxyribonucleic acid (DNA)—are the building blocks of all living organisms. They are responsible for storing your genetic info and contain all the instructions needed for your cells to develop and do their jobs.

Together, this Fantastic Four of macromolecules makes up the majority of the dry weight of every one of your cells—I say "dry" because your cells are also packed with water—and are responsible for a litany of jobs that dictate, direct, and manage your cells' functions. So you can only imagine how messing with any of these big four can completely f*ck up how well you age.

HOW MACROMOLECULES AFFECT YOUR AGE

What a half-century of research[1] has proven is that damage to proteins, DNA, lipids, and other molecular components within cells accumulates with age. The thing is, a screwed-up cell really isn't a big deal because your body tidies up after itself by eating the cell, breaking it down, and reusing the molecules for either energy or to make new cells. I know that sounds gross, but it's a good thing, a process called autophagy—telling that cell to self-destruct (apoptosis) to make room for a new cell.

Some cells, though, just don't know when or how to quit. Some old or damaged cells stop dividing but refuse to die, and instead enter a state known as cellular senescence. They basically become zombie cells, sitting inside your tissues waiting for something to put them out of their misery.

It's a protective mechanism meant to keep damaged cells from becoming cancerous, but it also prevents your old, worn-out tissues from replenishing themselves. Worse yet, these zombie cells secrete stuff that ages you faster, such as pro-inflammatory cytokines,[2] which damage healthier cells. For example, most skin cells produce collagen, but once they become senescent, they start producing collagenase, an enzyme that actually breaks down collagen, which may contribute to some of the wrinkling and thinning of your skin down the road.

The older you get, the more these zombie senescent cells can accumulate, thanks to a less than efficient autophagy process and immune system (among other things). Then your tissues and organs become filled with a bunch of uninvited walking dead cells, which is thought to contribute to a range of age-related diseases, from osteoarthritis to kidney dysfunction.

The fact is this: between repair problems, cellular death, and senescence, macromolecular damage helps drive the aging process. So what exactly is turning the screw on your cells? Oh, so many things. That constant beat-down can come from a variety of bullies, including the usual suspects you probably expect to hear about, such as toxins, cigarette smoke, and UV light, for example. But there are a few processes you can point a finger at that are critical to cellular carnage.

Mitochondrial dysfunction: One way aging starts to creep its way into your life is through your mitochondria, the tiny organelles inside your cells that act as their power source. They're the guys responsible for (among many tasks) converting nutrients into energy. However, many scientists believe that dysfunction of mitochondria is a big driver in aging.

When your mitochondria behave badly, it screws up other processes, from how well they communicate with your cell[3] to how much energy they produce. They can even cause inflammation, as well as make cells die before their time.[4] As a result, mitochondrial dysfunction contributes to various age-related conditions and diseases, such as cancer, heart disease, diabetes, and Alzheimer's.

Also, these little generators of energy create a natural by-product known as reactive oxygen species (ROS for short). These tiny molecules aren't all bad and actually help out in many areas, including supporting your immune system and helping cells communicate (more on that in a sec). But one type of ROS— free radicals—well, they're toxic and not so helpful.

So what exactly are free radicals? They're atoms, ions, or molecules that are unstable because they contain an unpaired electron. Electrons orbit around an atom, and as long as an atom has just the right number of electrons (and that number depends on the molecule in question), then everything's fine.

But when an atom is missing an electron, it becomes unstable, and these free radicals freak out and try to stabilize themselves by either stealing electrons from or giving them away to neighboring molecules. And trust me, free radicals are not choosy. They'll play the old electron switcheroo with any nearby molecule, whether it's a protein, lipid, carbohydrate, or DNA. When they do that, it damages that neighboring molecule by oxidizing it. Ever see a slice of apple turn brown? That apple is losing electrons. Now picture how losing electrons can damage a cell's DNA, structure, and ability to function.

So how does it get so out of control? As your mitochondria process nutrients, they need oxygen to convert food into energy, and the natural by-products of that cellular metabolism are free radicals. But your mitochondria aren't the only ones to blame. Everything from drugs to cigarette smoke, too much or too little oxygen, high sugar, too much exercise, pollutants, radiation, and other nasty external sources can expose you to these tiny, electron-deficient molecular thieves!

Typically, all those free radicals get neutralized by antioxidants produced by our cells. That's right—you make your own antioxidants. (You've probably heard about foods that also provide antioxidants, like blueberries or dark chocolate.) And what antioxidants do is basically find free radicals and give them an electron to shut them up and make them stable again. However, when free radicals dodge this cleanup and start piling up, oxidative stress—also known as oxidative damage—occurs, which is damage caused by an imbalance that allows too many free radicals to float around. Those extra free radicals can impair DNA, proteins, and mitochondria. Making matters worse, the more damage your mitochondria suffer, the more dysfunctional they become and the more free radicals they produce! So, you see, if you let things go with regard to your health, these body processes get out of control and it becomes an insane, vicious cycle.

Oxidative stress is believed by some to be a huge contributor to aging. But as it turns out, our understanding of free radicals may not be entirely complete when it comes to aging. Does oxidative stress rise as we age? Yes. Do antioxidant enzymes protect our cells? Hell, yes. But there's been a lot of research over the last decade showing that increasing antioxidants doesn't always affect our life expectancy.[5] Still, I think it's better to be safe than sorry. Plus, many of the foods that are rich in antioxidants—such as fruits and vegetables—are extremely healthy for many other reasons. So to not help your body out by fortifying yourself with the right amount of antioxidants, on the off chance that science may be wrong about them, makes no sense to me. That's why you'll see I'm all about getting as many antioxidants as possible through your diet.

Loss of proteostasis: Your proteins handle so many tasks, but in order for a protein molecule to do its job, it has to be folded perfectly into a specific, unique shape so that it can be identified and fully functional. Otherwise, it remains jobless and possibly destructive.

Inside your cells, proteins are constantly being assembled in a process called proteostasis. If a protein molecule looks like it just came back from the cleaner, all professionally laundered and perfectly creased, then it's recognized for what its job is and gets put to work.

But if it comes back looking distorted and messy, like your four-year-old folded it, then digestive enzymes called lysosomes gobble up that protein and break it down. If not for these lysosomes, that poor little misfolded protein would sit around without a job and perhaps start hanging out with other misshapen, jobless proteins — and that's when things can turn toxic or downright ugly in your cell.

If proteostasis becomes less efficient, you're eventually left with either too many or not enough proteins, a situation that studies[6] show contributes to many age-related issues, such as cataracts, diabetes, dilated cardiomyopathy, Alzheimer's disease, and Parkinson's.[7]

AGEs: Your macromolecules can also start bonding inappropriately with different macromolecules. As they get older, your proteins, DNA, and other structural molecules sometimes have a midlife crisis and hook up with others they shouldn't — something scientists call cross-linking. Once these unnecessary bonds form, the mobility and elasticity of the molecule decrease.

One of the main ways this happens is through a process called glycation, where sugar (glucose) molecules stick to a protein, lipid, or a nucleic acid, turning them into advanced glycosylation end products (or AGEs). When AGEs stick to neighboring macromolecules, they create a permanent link that shuts down that macromolecule's functions. This contributes to things like wrinkles, age-related cataracts, atherosclerosis, kidney decline, and the formation of beta-amyloid, the protein that clumps together in the brains of Alzheimer's patients.

Genomic instability: Your DNA has its own issues to worry about. Free-radical exposure, radiation (from X-rays or gamma rays, for example), toxins and chemicals, and glitches created when DNA replicates all cause cumulative damage over time.

Your cells have a system of repair mechanisms that do everything from reverse mistakes to rejoin broken DNA strands. But if
those systems fail, mutations pile up and turbo-charge aging[8] by
causing cell dysfunction and death.[9] Many age-related diseases
are linked with faulty DNA repair mechanisms, including
Alzheimer's, Parkinson's, and Lou Gehrig's disease (ALS).

Altered intercellular communication: Our cells can start to have problems speaking to each other. Well…not so much "speaking" as
"secreting" to each other (which really sounds disgusting, but
that's honestly how all of your cells communicate in order to grow
and function normally). They secrete signaling molecules to
neighboring cells, and they send molecular messengers through
your bloodstream to affect cells and tissues elsewhere in your
body.

The problem is, the older you get, the more difficult it becomes
for your cells to communicate. Your cells either start sending the
wrong messages to each other or the messages never get received—
a hot mess that prevents cells from growing and functioning normally. This impaired communication also keeps your immune
system from recognizing and removing damaged cells and pathogens, increasing your risk of many age-related infections, cancers, and other diseases.

New research[10] has shed light on why the immune system
weakens with age. It seems that immune cells in older tissues lose
coordination and become inconsistent in their ability to follow
directions. Picture your immune system like a cell army, ready to
protect the body from infection. When you're young, all your
cells work together to block pathogens, and it's that organization
that makes your immune system stronger. But as you get older,
that cell coordination breaks down. So instead of an army, your

immune system acts like some out-of-control PTA meeting where no one's listening to anyone else.

This is why an aging immune system is now considered one of the root causes of cancer and is the current focus of most anti-cancer efforts worldwide. When researchers[11] at the University of Dundee examined two million cases of more than one hundred different types of cancer among patients ages eighteen to seventy, they found an extremely strong link between the odds of cancer formation and the natural reduction of new T cells—a type of white blood cell that kills dysfunctional cells and foreign agents.

Stem cell exhaustion: But wait a minute. What about stem cells? Aren't they the answer to all this? After all, your stem cells exist in every part of your body and remain at the ready until they're needed to regenerate damaged tissues and replenish dying cells. They're the reason salamanders can grow back lopped-off legs and a zebra fish can replace pieces of its heart—they never run out of stem cells!

So here's how it works. There are three kinds of stem cells: embryonic, which help an embryo develop into a baby; induced pluripotent, stem cells made in laboratories; and adult, stem cells that exist in your brain, blood vessels, skin, heart, gut, and even your teeth! The number of stem cells you actually have in your body is anyone's guess, but they're rare. For example, according to the National Institutes of Health, only an estimated one in ten thousand to fifteen thousand cells in bone marrow is a stem cell.

Like lifeguards, stem cells basically sit and do nothing until there's a sudden need for more cells, either to maintain or to repair tissue due to injury or disease. When that happens, the stem cells in that damaged area start dividing, and each new cell has the potential to either remain a stem cell or become something completely different—such as a red blood cell, a muscle cell, or even a brain cell—depending on where it's located.

But there are a few catches. You only have a limited amount of stem cells in each location, and once they are used up, that's it. They're like dollars on a gift card—use them all up and eventually your body has nothing to spend. This is called stem cell exhaustion—and it sucks. Plus, stem cells are not invincible! They are just like any other cell, in that they are susceptible to things like DNA damage, mitochondrial dysfunction, and cellular senescence.

Science has identified stem cell therapy as a game-changer that could radically transform how we treat age-related disease. Right now, scientists are attempting to use bone marrow stem cells to rejuvenate ovaries[12]—allowing them to produce more estrogen in young women that suffer from premature ovarian insufficiency—and to reverse macular degeneration[13] via a stem-cell patch implant. They've even recently figured out how to reprogram skin cells into stem cells by activating a particular gene[14] (in mice, for now). But even though several stem cell treatments already exist—such as bone marrow transplants for leukemia—stem cell transplantation isn't as easy as it sounds.

First off, stem cells are not magic—they can only turn into the type of tissue they came from. In other words, you can't just take a stem cell found in fat and use it to replace stem cells in your heart or liver—it doesn't work like that. Also, transplanting healthy lab-grown stem cells into damaged or disease-ridden areas isn't easy because your immune system's first instinct is to reject the transplant. Scientists are looking into ways to modify stem cells in the lab using gene therapy and other techniques to overcome this immune rejection, but we're not quite there yet.

Even the National Institutes of Health[15] says, and I quote: "Stem cells offer exciting promise for future therapies, but significant technical hurdles remain that will only be overcome through years of intensive research." So don't believe the hype that fly-by-night clinics promising stem cell miracles may be pitching you. But it's also okay to get excited about the future. With more than one thousand stem cell–related clinical trials happening out there, there may be something to talk about soon.

By the way, what about umbilical cord blood? Isn't that stuff pumped full of stem cells—and could it help your child live a lot longer one day? If you had a doctor clamp your baby's umbilical cord to collect some blood that's now stored at a cord blood bank—or if you are just thinking about it—know this: scientists have been able to rejuvenate the memory and brain performance of old mice by around 30 to 50 percent using injections of cord blood from humans, due in part to a protein (TIMP2) that's abundant in cord blood but diminishes as we age. But those are mice—and it wasn't the stem cells but the protein that helped. On top of that, no one really knows how long frozen cord blood really lasts because it's such a new thing. Current research says that stored blood is only useful for up to fifteen years, so if you're thinking it may help your kid live longer down the road, know that it will probably be expired before they even see their first wrinkle.

WHAT THE FUTURE HOLDS

Science is still unclear on whether macromolecular damage causes aging or aging causes macromolecular damage. Regardless, it's a vicious cycle that feeds on itself, and that's why researchers are trying to manipulate your macromolecules to reverse aging.

Connect and conquer: One mind-blowing possibility is parabiosis[16]—the surgical joining of two organisms. In one study, for example,[17] researchers surgically linked the circulatory systems of two mice (one old and one young) to mix their blood. After four weeks, the old mouse's thick, hypertrophied heart was healthy again, thanks to a protein more commonly found in the blood of young mice called growth differentiation factor 11 (or GDF11).

Right now, the most promising research in parabiosis shows that a patient's own plasma might help heal wounds, regenerate tissue, and potentially reverse some age-related factors. In fact, researchers[18] have already discovered that giving old mice the umbilical cord plasma of human fetuses makes them faster learners by enhancing activity in their hippocampi, the brain regions behind learning and memory. However, further studies are required to see if swapping blood could have any effect on humans.

Have a DNA do-over: Reversing cellular aging by fixing your DNA is another area of interest. Researchers are exploring a wide variety of options, ranging from controlling an RNA molecule named Zeb2-NAT (which seems to rejuvenate old cells in mice)[19] to using a synthetic molecule called PIP-S2 that binds with DNA and has been shown to regenerate heart muscle cells in twelve days.[20]

One compound, nicotinamide mononucleotide (NMN), seems to boost nicotinamide adenine dinucleotide (NAD+), a metabolite found in every cell that plays a big part in regulating the interactions that control DNA repair and that decline with age. When researchers[21] at the University of New South Wales treated mice with NMN, it quickly improved their cells' ability to repair DNA damage caused by radiation exposure and old age. It's been shown to be so effective that NASA thinks it may allow astronauts to get to Mars!

Upgrade your cellular network: Other scientists are working on finding a way to activate all those senescent zombie cells. A study[22] out of the University of Exeter found that some types of genes (known as splicing factors) become gradually dormant as we age. But by applying resveratrol—a compound found naturally in red grapes, wine, dark chocolate, and blueberries—to cells in culture, those genes become active again! Within hours, the cells started to act like young cells by dividing and lengthening their telomeres (a key I explain in chapter 9).

Science is also looking at eliminating those zombie cells using senolytics, an emerging type of drug that seems to be successful in clearing them out and alleviating a range of age- and disease-related problems in other species. One example is the drug rapamycin, an immunosuppressant primarily used in organ transplants that seems to stimulate cellular recycling (autophagy) and to extend the life span of mice. Rapamycin has also been shown[23] to prevent age-related loss of stem cells in flies and mice.

Another is metformin, one of the most common anti-diabetes drugs in the United States, which is already known to increase the amount of toxic oxygen molecules released within a cell. For some strange reason, even though this should be bad for your cells, it actually seems to make them stronger, slowing down the aging process and extending the life span of worms and mice.[24]

Some scientists are going right to the heart of the problem. A team at the Albert Einstein College of Medicine[25] is fiddling with stem cells in the hypothalamus (a part of the brain that regulates the automatic nervous system, which handles functions like regulating body temperature, monitoring hunger, and prompting sleep) to see if life span could be extended that way. These hypothalamic stem cells release molecules called microRNAs (miRNAs) that help regulate your genes. When they injected miRNAs directly into middle-aged mice whose stem cells had been destroyed, they significantly slowed the aging process while also improving coordination, muscle endurance, cognitive ability, and even social behavior.

Tired of collecting too many free radicals? University of Michigan researchers[26] are hard at work looking for ways to stimulate lysosomes, proteins that act as powerful protectants against free radicals and oxidative stress. Sick of your immune system doing a half-ass job? Right now, it's thought[27] that SIRT1 — an anti-aging protein in cells that is activated by resveratrol — could be used to rejuvenate mature T cells, which can become toxic as you age.

Con your cells: The final exciting thing science might pull off one day is stripping faulty mitochondria from your cells before they screw sh*t up in the first place. A team led by Newcastle University found[28] that when they tricked aging cells into eliminating defective mitochondria—a process known as mitophagy—levels of oxygen free radicals and inflammatory molecules returned to those of younger cells.

WHAT WE KNOW NOW

Even though the greatest minds on Earth will admit they are perpetually scratching their heads for all the answers, there is a lot that we do know now and a lot we can do about aging.

What to Eat

I take that back—make that "what not to eat." I say that because one of the biggest areas of interest in geroscience right now is the impact of calorie restriction on both extending life span *and* health span—the amount of time you stay healthy.

By the way: whenever I mention calorie restriction (or CR) and throw out percentages indicating how much participants have reduced their calorie intake, you're probably asking, how many calories does that even mean? What's the starting point? In pretty much every study that talks about calorie restriction and aging, the percentages of restriction are revealed but not the actual calorie counts because the starting point can vary from person to person. I've seen studies that had participants record what they ate for up to a month; then from there, the scientists figured out what their average calorie intake was on a daily basis and used that number as their standard daily calorie requirement. I've also seen studies that used a person's basal metabolic rate (BMR)—the number of calories needed to keep your body functioning at rest—as the starting point. When it comes to aging research, one thing's for sure: the subjects in these studies are always eating less than they have historically.

The key is to find the balance between calorie deprivation (starving your body of essential macro- and micronutrients) and calorie restriction. Not to worry—I spell out exactly how to find your ideal calorie allowance for optimal health and longevity in chapter 13.

Could fasting "speed up" your stem cells?

You've got stem cells everywhere, including your gut. That's right, you actually have intestinal stem cells that continuously renew themselves. But over time, they start to lose their ability to regenerate, which can set you down the path of being more susceptible to gastrointestinal infections and other intestinal-based issues. However, scientists think there's a way to jump-start those stem cells by merely stepping back from eating for a day.

According to a new study[29] out of MIT, the cells of mice that fasted for twenty-four hours began to use fatty acids over glucose for energy. This change from burning carbohydrates to burning fat seemed to stimulate the intestinal stem cells, making them more regenerative. When researchers removed and examined their stem cells, they noticed that the fasting mice had doubled their regenerative capability.

Ultimately, eating less food has been shown to be effective at reversing many age-related issues in a variety of organisms — not just us. Eating less has helped mice live 40 percent longer and monkeys more than 20 percent longer.[30] You'll soon hear about how calorie restriction influences many of the 6 Keys. But for now, here's what eating less does for your macromolecules (as long as you're still getting everything your body needs nutritionally).

A recent two-year study[31] out of the School of Public Health at Georgia State University found that when participants reduced their daily calories by 25 percent, they had fewer signs of oxidative stress than participants who ate as they pleased. But that's not all. Calorie restriction has been shown to improve mitochondrial function and reduce DNA/RNA damage in adults and to lower your risk of cardiovascular disease.[32]

As for fighting off free radicals, your body naturally produces antioxidants (glutathione peroxidase, for example) to protect against oxidative damage. Getting antioxidants through your diet doesn't hurt, but don't focus just on the ones you *think* are more important, such as vitamin C and vitamin E, for example.

Your best bet is to eat the widest variety of fruits and vegetables possible. Not because you have to ingest every single vitamin and mineral, but because fruits and vegetables actually increase your production of glutathione peroxidase and resistance to oxidation more efficiently[33] than popping a supplement containing the same exact vitamins and minerals.

That doesn't mean there aren't a few nutrients you should take, but it's always important to fire on all cylinders. For example, according to a new study[34] out of University of Texas at Arlington's College of Nursing and Health Innovation, zinc seems to selectively stop the growth of esophageal cancer cells. In addition, omega-3 supplementation has been proven to reduce oxidative stress by about 15 percent.[35]

Vitamin C may also be able to do more than just boost your immune system. Researchers[36] from NYU Langone's Perlmutter Cancer Center believe that the vitamin may also help kill older, damaged stem cells found in bone marrow by activating an enzyme called TET2. Without that enzyme, those faulty stem cells multiply into even more faulty stem cells, which can contribute to certain blood cancers.

Another way to maintain your macromolecules is by keeping your cytokines under control. These proteins act as chemical messengers that regulate your immune response to infection, but when they linger, they can also become pro-inflammatory and cause tissue damage.[37] If you're getting enough omega-3s and eating eight or more servings of vegetables daily, you're already reducing the concentration of "bad" cytokines significantly. But shying away from saturated fats, avoiding trans fats altogether, and sticking with polyunsaturated fats seems to lower[38] pro-inflammatory cytokines as well.

You can also do something about advanced glycosylation end products, or AGEs (these little buggers stick to neighboring macromolecules, creating a permanent link that shuts down that macromolecule's functions): avoid processed foods and sugar as much as possible—the less sugar you eat, the less sugar is floating in your bloodstream for proteins and fats to cling to. Even foods from animal sources (pork, beef, fish, chicken, and even eggs) naturally contain AGEs.

On their own, animal-based foods aren't that bad since your body can process AGEs. But how you cook these foods[39] really matters. When meat is cooked at a higher, drier temperature (such as by grilling, frying, baking, or broiling), it causes even more AGEs to form. Research has shown that cooking those same foods using moist heat for shorter cooking times and at lower temperatures seems to produce fewer AGEs, making steaming, stewing, or boiling better options.

But if you're not into boiled chicken breast, first off, welcome to the club! Second, just minimizing how often you cook with high, dry heat and using a few tricks can help. For example, exposing meat to radiant rather than direct heat works best. (That means no sticking it right under the broiler or over the coals/fire.) Also, marinating your meat gives it more moisture during the cooking process. Your smartest option: use vinegar, lemon juice, or tomato juice, since acidic ingredients have the antioxidants that decrease the production of AGEs.

Finally, remember what I told you about protein being a major player in your cells? Getting enough protein in your diet is important, and new data explains that it's also critical to space out protein consumption evenly throughout the day. When research-ers[40] at McGill University Health Centre in Quebec followed 1,800 people between the ages of sixty-seven and eighty-four for three years, they found that participants who had consumed pro-tein in a balanced way throughout the day had greater muscle mass and strength than those who consumed more during the evening and less at breakfast.

How to Sweat

We've known for a while that regular exercise seems to reduce AGEs; that low-volume, high-intensity intervals increase muscle mitochondrial capacity in patients with type-2 diabetes; and that endurance training triggers systemic mitochondrial rejuvenation in mice.[41] But the latest news about the age-defying effects of high-intensity interval training (HIIT) may be the breakthrough your cells have been waiting for.

A recent study[42] took two groups of volunteers—half between the ages of eighteen and thirty and the other half between the ages of sixty-five and eighty—and had them perform three dif-ferent exercise programs: high-intensity interval biking, strength training with weights, and strength training/interval training. Then they took biopsies from their thigh muscles and compared their cells to those of sedentary participants.

Although strength training helped build muscle mass, HIIT had the biggest impact on the cellular level, boosting mitochon-drial capacity in the younger group by 49 percent and in the older group by a whopping 69 percent—all while improving their insulin sensitivity and stimulating the production of ribosomes, which are responsible for producing your cells' protein building blocks. However, HIIT wasn't as effective as strength training at building muscle strength, which typically drops as we age. Therefore, incorporating both HIIT and strength training can cover all bases.

Now here's the thing about exercise—it's also a source of oxidative stress and increases levels of free radicals in your system. That should make sense, right? If your mitochondria are working even harder to generate the energy you need to power through your workout, and a by-product of all that effort is an increase in free radicals, then the more you push yourself, the more oxidative stress you're causing.

But guess what? Regular exercise simultaneously reduces oxidative stress by increasing antioxidant production.[43] In fact, the more you exercise, the more antioxidants your body produces. Studies have shown that even the brief, sudden rise in free radicals created from exercise not only elevates antioxidants, but also triggers a few metabolic processes that make you even more resistant to oxidative stress.

But what about extreme bouts of exercise? I mean, exercise *has* to be just like everything else in life—if you push things too far, you pay for it later, right? Well, it turns out that the key factor in how much oxidative damage you're causing when you work out is not determined by how much you exercise, but by whether your body is ready for what you're throwing at it.

No matter how hard you train and no matter what activity you do (running, strength training, cycling, whatever), so long as you're smart about not pushing yourself beyond your limits, your body will naturally adjust and increase your antioxidant levels to match.

However, if you don't train consistently or know your limits, your antioxidant system never gets the chance to build up and prepare itself for the oxidative stress that exercise causes. In other words, if you only exercise sporadically, push yourself too hard before you're ready to handle a higher training volume, or never give your body enough time to recover, your antioxidant system won't ever become strong enough to keep up and prevent oxidative damage. But if you exercise on a regular basis and raise the intensity, length, and frequency of your workouts only when your body's ready for it, science says you'll be just fine.

What to Watch For

Some of the well-known ways to avoid damage to your macromolecules still hold true, such as reducing your exposure to the sun (and radiation in general), air pollutants, alcohol, and cigarette smoke.[44]

But even the simplest of choices—such as burning the candle at both ends—can screw with you. In fact, just one night of partial sleep deprivation promotes[45] biological aging. When participants were asked to switch from sleeping a full eight hours (11:00 p.m. to 7:00 a.m.) to sleeping from 3:00 a.m. to 7:00 a.m., their blood revealed changes consistent with an increase in the DNA-damage response and cell senescence.

If you manage to go to bed on time, even the light you're exposed to beforehand could be affecting your molecules in mysterious ways. In a recent study,[46] when hamsters didn't receive a natural mix of daylight and darkness before mating, their pups were born with weakened immune systems. It's a discovery that researchers say builds a strong case for putting down your cell phone early in the evening to reduce your exposure to dim light at night, since this disrupts melatonin in both rodents and humans and could impair how quickly your body heals. Less sleep equals less healing time anyway, so your immune system could be getting a double whammy every time you end the night staring at a screen.

CHAPTER 5

The Second Key: Engineering Epigenetics

Your DNA may take a beating as time passes, but here's the deal: even if you could keep every single double helix inside your body blissful and bulletproof from damage, something else can mess with your DNA in a different way.

Scientists now believe that several factors can actually *change* your genetic code. Scary, right? In fact, the lifestyle choices and experiences of your parents, grandparents, and great-grandparents, as well as exposure to processed food, smoking, and disease, can change your genetic traits in a way that not only brings on age-related issues but makes it possible for you to pass on those age-accelerating glitches to your kids.

It works like this: inside almost every cell in your body lies a genome, which is another name for a complete set of all of your twenty-thousand-plus genes. Each of your thirty-seven-trillion-plus cells contains all of the instructions on how to build and maintain, well, you! And every one of those cells is exactly alike.

So if the genetic info in every cell throughout your body is the same, how do your cells know what to become? In other words, how does a cell know whether it should be a bone cell, liver cell, muscle cell, brain cell, or a heart cell, for example? That's the role of the epigenome, a collection of chemical compounds and proteins that sort of sit on top of your DNA and decide each cell's job and function.

The epigenome is basically the boss that tells a cell what it should be by either turning on (activating) a few genes inside that cell or turning them off (keeping them dormant). How it takes control is by chemically modifying your DNA, or what's called marking the genome. These epigenetic marks don't damage your DNA. Instead, they merely tell the DNA inside a cell exactly what to do, when to do it, and where to do it.

Picture it this way: Your body needs a cell to be a skin cell. That cell has big dreams and could be anything it wants to be. But your epigenome steps in like an overbearing parent, turns on a few genes (the ones needed to turn that cell into a skin cell), then tells every other gene that might cause that cell to turn into anything else, "Don't even think about it!"

Just by suppressing or enhancing certain genes, the epigenome causes that cell to flip to the "How to Be a Good Little Skin Cell" chapter in your DNA's instruction manual, do everything by the book, and grow up to become exactly what your body needs it to be. Once a cell knows its job, it holds those epigenetic alterations every time it divides. So that skin cell stays a skin cell for life.

Your epigenome marks, or designates, your DNA in several ways, but to keep things simple, here are the big two. The first— *histone modification*—is the one that's a lot more fun to visualize. Inside the nucleus of every cell, there's a mass of genetic material called *chromatin,* made up of both DNA and histone proteins. It's where your DNA lives until it's time for a cell to divide. When that time comes, chromatin's main job is to compress your DNA into chromosomes so that everything fits nice and snug within the nucleus. It's sort of the scaffolding that keeps everything sorted and packed up for when the cell divides.

Anyway, those histone proteins also have tails, and your epigenome allows chemicals to bond with those tails, which change how tightly or loosely wound your DNA stays wrapped. By squeezing tightly, some genes get choked off, making them less accessible to proteins and harder to read by a cell—so those genes never get expressed. When histones relax, your DNA becomes more accessible to various proteins and your genes easier to read, allowing them to be expressed.

When everything is working properly, the tail is choking off portions and being relaxed with others to ensure that particular genes are active and others are contained. But, when it's not working properly, which can happen when chromatin doesn't do its job of regulating histones properly, it may be tightening things that shouldn't be tightened and loosening up on things that shouldn't be loosened. #CellularAnarchy—kidding. Sorta.

The second way your DNA is modified is through *DNA methylation*—when a molecule (called a methyl group) gets added to specific portions of your DNA to lock random genes into their off position. DNA methylation is important because it prevents genes from expressing themselves. Can you imagine if every gene in your body was turned on at once and every single process and genetic thing about you occurred simultaneously? It wouldn't be pretty.

Your cells wouldn't have any idea what their job was, when to stop growing, or what type of cell they should turn into! Beyond triggering countless mutations throughout your entire body, it would also mean that every gene that makes you predisposed to a specific disease, allergy, or life-threatening illness would also be active—all at the same time.

Anyway, when a methyl group gets added to a DNA molecule, it prevents that gene from turning on either by recruiting proteins involved in gene repression or by keeping a particular segment (or segments) of your DNA from being copied and proteins from being processed.

When it's humming along perfectly, it's all good. But when the process of methylation gets interfered with in a way that turns certain genes off that should remain on—which can happen as a result of genetic mutations or environmental risk factors—that's when things can start getting messed up.

HOW YOUR EPIGENETICS AFFECT YOUR AGE

The epigenetic changes that occur with aging are under constant study, and there are a few things science has figured out.

When you're young and healthy, all of these biological processes are precisely regulated within your cells (for the most part). But as the years fly by, your epigenome begins to change, and its ability to maintain itself starts to falter, causing it to make poorer decisions in the switch-flipping department—decisions that ultimately affect how your cells function on a molecular level.

Over time, random mistakes begin to occur as cells divide. Instead of splitting into two perfect copies of their mother cell, you're left with two daughter cells that aren't quite like their mama; they've either picked up a few bad habits (added a few epigenetic marks) or forgotten what their mom tried to teach them (lost a few epigenetic marks).

These mistakes can cause proteins to appear in cells where they shouldn't be and to disappear in cells where they are vital to survival. This is called epigenetic drift, and scientists feel it contributes to a variety of aging-related issues.

For instance, epigenetic drift can cause immune cells to suddenly forget what their job is; your immune system then weakens and leaves you less resilient to pathogens. Even muscle cells can be deactivated. This not only causes you to lose muscle, but also increases your risk of heart failure and other cardiovascular diseases, such as atherosclerosis.[1]

In addition, hypermethylation can occur, causing genes responsible for repairing DNA or suppressing tumors[2] to switch off. This is why it's now thought that epigenetics plays a major role in the development of certain cancers, such as stomach, kidney, and colon cancer.

The flipside is that over time your epigenome can also cause the removal of methyl groups from portions of your DNA (demethylation), switching on genes that should stay off. This can affect the stability of your genome, and decreased stability has also been linked to cancer, age-related bone loss, and possibly Alzheimer's disease.[3]

When DNA methylation becomes erratic, the same age-related changes start happening to your histones,[4] which can loosen or tighten the packaging of your DNA. Depending on whether they decide to give your DNA a firm or limp handshake, they can cause a variety of genes to get turned on or off,[5] for better or worse. Finally, epigenetics can also create problems for your chromatin. As you age, your cells become less efficient at chromatin remodeling, allowing for potential mutation of your DNA.

WHAT THE FUTURE HOLDS

Something you can't control, for now, is damage done to your epigenome courtesy of your family history. When you were conceived, you got one copy of genes from your mom and one copy from your dad, and, supposedly, a complete reset of the epigenome—a process known as reprogramming. What this means is that you get a clean copy of their genes that's free of any of the epigenomic changes that may have occurred throughout their entire lifetimes.

This process is supposed to ensure you get a fresh start instead of paying for the mistakes of your parents. But guess what? Scientists[6] think it might be possible to pass down epigenetic changes, *if* they happen in sperm or egg cells.[7] In fact, the tadpole and egg may avoid the reprogramming process altogether and pass down problems from one generation to the next.

For example, would you be shocked to know people who had been in utero during the Dutch famine of 1944 to 1945 were found to be heavier and more obese in adulthood,[8] making them more susceptible to chronic disease? And studies now show that the strength of your bones may be decided before you even have them. Researchers[9] at the University of Southampton found that women who had higher levels of methylation had children with less total bone mass.

Most recently, a group of researchers[10] at the University of Melbourne did a first-of-its-kind investigation of hundreds of people from twenty-five families that had multiple incidences of breast cancer: they found twenty-four previously unidentified epigenetic changes that alter a woman's risk of breast cancer—changes that are passed down through generations.

Most people think that because breast cancer runs in their

family, they must have some kind of mutation that was passed down. Researchers now believe that your genes could be absolutely fine. Instead, it could be that DNA methylation is heritable and can mimic genetic variation. And if they're right, this could open the door to treating and preventing a lot of heritable age-related illnesses and issues down the road.

While this news can seem a bit discouraging, here's the thing: you have the ability to fight your genetics. For example, while my metabolism is naturally slow—I was an overweight kid, my dad is overweight, and other members of his family are overweight—I have managed those genetics with deliberate actions that help me prevent becoming overweight and unhealthy. I eat clean. I don't overeat. I exercise, etc.

Conversely, this can also work in your favor. It used to be thought that the children of Holocaust survivors had an increased risk of PTSD and other mood and anxiety issues. But research[11] now shows that children of traumatized parents may have lower levels of methylation and seem to inherit traits that promote resilience as well as vulnerability to these disorders. New data[12] has even suggested that events that took place in the lives of our ancestors possibly as far back as fourteen generations could affect our overall development, altering our gene expression and DNA.

What gets the scientific community excited though is that what may be aging us is a bunch of genes all flipped in the wrong direction! They know that eventually we will be able to map out every gene and figure out how to prevent epigenetic alterations from screwing around with our switches. Then everything could potentially stay running smoothly indefinitely. Through simply taking control of one's epigenome, we could put an end to countless diseases, cancers, and even the process of aging itself.

Right now, scientists are hard at work figuring out how we

might be able to control or reverse epigenetic drift. For example, the Cancer Genome Atlas[13]—a collaboration of the National Cancer Institute and the National Human Genome Research Institute—is comparing the genomes and epigenomes of normal cells to those of cancer cells. Their goal: to try to map out all of the epigenomic changes that happen in DNA and cause cells to grow uncontrolled in an effort to one day detect, treat, and possibly prevent all two-hundred-plus forms of cancer. They have already generated comprehensive, multidimensional maps of the key genomic changes in thirty-three types of cancer thus far. How's that for crazy awesome and exciting?

What else is on the horizon? Researchers are exploring every inch of the epigenetic landscape to try to develop pharmaceuticals that may alter whatever is sending mixed messages to your genes. It's an adventure they foresee not only reversing aging and age-related disorders such as Alzheimer's, macular degeneration, high cholesterol, and type-2 diabetes, but also potentially stopping a whole host of issues ranging from neurodevelopmental disorders and viruses to obesity and even addiction.

Science is already having success editing genomes, adding and removing methyl groups, and essentially reversing diseases in mice using a technology called CRISPR-Cas9.[14] This system creates a small piece of RNA that attaches to a designated spot on your genome and cuts your DNA at that precise location. As your cell starts immediately repairing the damage, scientists use that window of time before it's completely healed to access whichever genes may need to be flipped back on or off in that location.

Further study is being focused on how to use epigenetics to refresh your skin cells. Researchers[15] from the Perelman School of Medicine at the University of Pennsylvania recently found that a key protein called KMT2D is a crucial coordinator during our skin's turnover process. The hope? That a topical therapy might one day be developed to prevent and treat skin cancer.

Sounds like science fiction, right? As I mentioned, we aren't there yet. And even if we were, I wouldn't want you relying solely on external solutions. I need you empowered and proactive. So let's jump into what you can do right now.

WHAT WE KNOW NOW

It turns out your environment[16]—what you eat and drink, how you exercise, and what you're exposed to—has a huge influence on your epigenome and how you age. There are several ways to get an edge over your epigenetics.

What to Eat

In addition to all its other benefits, calorie restriction has been shown to delay age-related methylation. When investigators at the Lewis Katz School of Medicine at Temple University[17] reduced calorie intake by 30 percent in monkeys, they noticed significant reductions in epigenetic drift and found that the monkeys displayed a blood-methylation age equivalent to animals seven years younger.

It's not just how much you eat, but what you throw back[18] that keeps your epigenome nice and happy. For example, you need to moderate your fat consumption—period! It turns out binging on high-fat meals—even in the short term[19]—can cause widespread DNA methylation changes[20] that may affect close to 45 percent of your genes (primarily those involved in inflammation, the reproductive system, and cancer).

Now, I'm betting this one confused you as much as it initially confused me, because these days we hear constantly that good fats are healthy for you. The key here is good fats *in moderation*. And not to worry, I map out all the guidelines for you in the 6 Keys strategy. The main takeaway in terms of improving epigenetics is that monounsaturated and omega–3 fats are best (the type of fats commonly found in foods such as olive oil or salmon, for example), but not too much of them, and trans and saturated fats should be avoided or restricted whenever possible.

A few foods in particular are seriously DNA-friendly. One of them is green tea, which is rich in epigallocatechin-3-gallate, a compound that may[21] help keep DNA methylation in check. Even though scientists have not identified exactly how the compounds in green tea subdue DNA methylation, they continue to examine how green tea might create epigenetic changes that could prevent cancer.[22] Sidenote: when you drink it, be sure it's organic and NOT decaffeinated, since some of green tea's healthy compounds get destroyed during the decaffeination process.

Cruciferous vegetables such as cauliflower, kale, broccoli, Brussels sprouts, cabbage, rutabaga, Chinese cabbage, bok choy, turnips, collards, radishes, arugula, and watercress are also epigenome-friendly. They contain isothiocyanates, which help your histones do their job, as well as natural folate, a key vitamin used in DNA methylation.[23] Studies have shown that when you are running low on folate and your cells divide, the production of an enzyme known as thymidine can be compromised. When that happens, your body makes a substitution and uses a compound called uracil instead in the DNA sequence. This may cause your DNA to attempt to repair the defect, which increases your risk of chromosomal breaks.

When in doubt about which cruciferous vegetables to eat, go for the dark, leafy, green veggies, which tend to be richer in vitamins and minerals. Just be sure to consume them cooked instead of raw as often as possible to avoid excess goitrogens, substances that can disrupt thyroid function. Once cooked (just throwing them in a pot of boiling water for a few minutes, draining them, then patting them down to dry them off will do the trick), most of the goitrogens become deactivated.

Foods rich in B vitamins (especially B6 and B12)[24] such as salmon, spinach, and avocados, for example, also give your body what it needs to keep your DNA methylation running smoothly. New research out of Nova Southeastern University in Fort Lauderdale has shown that vitamin B12 levels in the brain decline with age. On average, older individuals between the ages of sixty-one and eighty were observed to have three times less B12 in their brains than younger individuals. Even worse, older people were also found to have ten times less methylcobalamin (methyl B12) than younger people. Methyl B12 is an active form of the vitamin that supports normal brain development through the regulation of gene expression. Scientists think it's that massive drop that could adversely disrupt learning and memory as we get older.

Finally, adding the right spices seems to pay off. For example, curcumin, a compound found in turmeric, has been shown to have multiple positive effects on your genes by impacting your DNA.[25] Many studies have revealed curcumin's importance in regulating the expression of important genes by reversing DNA methylation and altering histone modifications. Curcumin helps reduce[26] the risk of age-related diseases, including cancer, diabetic nephropathy, and neurocognitive disorders such as Alzheimer's disease.

How to Sweat

I know you know exercise is good for you, but did you know it goes genes deep? In one landmark study[27] from the Karolinska Institute in Sweden, it was found that long-term endurance training for forty-five minutes, four times a week created new gene patterns within muscle tissue after three months—patterns that had a positive effect on insulin response, inflammation, and energy metabolism. In that short amount of time, endurance training had affected an average of more than five thousand DNA methylation sites on the genome of muscle cells.

Ever heard the term muscle memory? Well, it's a real thing and your epigenome is the key. A recent study[28] by researchers at Keele University found that some genes get marked—or unmarked—after a muscle grows from resistance training. Because of this, whenever you take time off from exercise, it's these markings that may be behind a muscle having a greater response to exercise when you start training those muscles. So if you've ever worked out but haven't in a while, know this: your genes are at the ready, so that when you start exercising again, they are designed to build themselves back up faster and stronger than the first time you trained them as a beginner. And if you've never exercised before, it's time to start marking up your epigenome!

Getting your fitness in also affects your fat cells. Researchers at Lund University in Sweden found[29] that even two exercise sessions a week can cause genome-wide positive changes in DNA methylation within adipose (fat) tissue. When they looked specifically at genes linked to type-2 diabetes and obesity, they found altered DNA methylation. In English, this means that physical activity affects genes in a way that lowers your risk for many age-related diseases. I know... shocker, but still, it's always important to remember why you put in the work.

Amazingly, just one single exercise session has been proven[30] to cause immediate changes in the methylation pattern of a variety of different genes—*one!* Even better, the older you are, the more exercise seems[31] to improve methylation. So it's never too late to use exercise to keep your DNA functioning properly.

On the other hand, blowing off exercise is the worst thing you can do for your epigenetics. In one large-scale international study that looked at the effects of a high BMI (body mass index) on the genome, scientists examined the blood samples of more than ten thousand European men and women. The study—the world's largest[32] of its kind—discovered that a high BMI epigenetically altered 207 different genes and significantly changed the expression of genes responsible for lipid metabolism and inflammation. What that means is that by simply sitting around, you'll be marking your epigenome in a way that interferes with your body's ability to convert fats into energy and ratchets up inflammation—and trust me, as you'll soon know, you definitely don't want to do that.

What to Watch For

On top of proper diet and exercise, here's a hard-and-fast rule: if it's known to be toxic, poisonous, or bad for you in general, it's probably making methylation alterations that are definitely not helping you age any slower.

Some of your epigenome's primary enemies include the soot in air pollution, asbestos, and low levels of benzene (an industrial solvent found in paint, detergents, varnish, glue, pesticides, industrial cleaners, gas, and other fuels—and even in dryer sheets and paraffin wax candles!)

But wait folks, that's not all. Other insidious gene abusers are two obvious culprits: too much sun and smoking. New findings show that the impact of smoking is longer-lasting than previously thought when it comes to your epigenetics. When researchers[33] compared the blood samples of nearly sixteen thousand current and former smokers, they noticed a few frightening facts.

DNA methylation sites connected with smoking were discovered on more than seven thousand genes—that means smoking affects one third of your genes! In former smokers, some of those DNA methylation sites remain affected for well beyond thirty years. The good news is that once you quit, the majority of those sites return to the same levels as a nonsmoker within five years, appearing as if they were never affected in the first place.

There are two additional chemicals of note that can wreak havoc on your epigenome: bisphenol A and phthalates. Bisphenol A (BPA) hides in canned foods as well as products like food storage containers, water bottles, and polycarbonate tableware. Food can absorb this compound, which may accelerate the aging process[34] and put you at greater risk of atherosclerosis-related disease.

And if you needed another reason to shy away from BPA, then do it for your kids. It's been shown[35] that exposure to the chemical triggers epigenetic changes associated with adult-onset disease that can be passed on to future generations (what is known as transgenerational epigenetic inheritance). So the sooner you avoid BPA, the longer you'll live—and the same goes for anyone you end up giving life to down the road.

As for phthalates, they are found in everything from insect repellent to nail polish, carpeting, shower curtains, vinyl flooring, and almost anything scented, such as air fresheners, laundry detergent, and even shampoos. This chemical is just as guilty of tweaking methylation in ways that can trigger a series of adverse health effects such as immune disorders, cancer, and diabetes.[36] To top it all off, being around all that smelly stuff even makes your muscles weaker.

In a study[37] of more than twelve hundred people (men and women with an average age of about seventy-five), researchers found an inverse relationship between the subject's hand strength and the levels of phthalates in their urine. You may not care — I mean, so what? My hair smells nicer at the expense of a weaker handshake? But previous studies have reported that hand strength is a good measure of whole-body strength,[38] and a weaker grip is associated with cognitive deterioration, functional disability, and increased mortality[39] — so there's that!

Now, if you're wondering, "What the hell am I supposed to do with all this overwhelming info?" not to worry. Remember, this has all been integrated into a strategy so that you don't have to try to figure it out on your own. Cool? Good.

You're not antisocial — it's your epigenome

Social engagement has positive effects on your health and longevity, and conversely, prolonged isolation has been shown to be a greater health hazard than obesity[40] and as strong of a risk factor for early mortality as smoking nearly fifteen cigarettes a day. But could the reason you're not as social have to do with DNA methylation?

When researchers[41] looked at the DNA samples of more than 120 volunteers, they found that when OXT genes (the ones responsible for the "love hormone," oxytocin) were affected due to higher levels of methylation, participants had a harder time recognizing emotional facial expressions, which can impede your ability to form healthy relationships and be more empathetic. Participants were also more likely to be more anxious in their relationships with loved ones. The more elevated their levels of methylation, the lower their levels of oxytocin.

Hold a baby — and you may help them age slower!

According to new data[42] from the University of British Columbia and the BC Children's Hospital Research Institute, the amount of time you spend in close and comforting contact with babies affects them on a molecular level for up to four years. When researchers looked at the levels of DNA methylation among children who had experienced more distress and less physical contact as a baby, there was a noticeable epigenetic difference in five specific DNA sites, particularly in genes related to both their metabolism and their immune system.

CHAPTER 6

The Third Key: Strong-Arming Stress

We've all seen presidents leave office with gray hair and sunken faces, looking twice as old as when they started. We've all known people that have gone through hard times or worked demanding jobs who seem to come out the other end riddled with excess wrinkles, eye bags, thinning hair, and a host of other symptoms that come with premature aging.

So why does this happen? First we need to understand what stress actually is—and how it affects our physiology. Then we can tackle how to combat it. So don't let this chapter stress you out. Bad pun, I know, but help is on the way.

So, what is stress? I'm guessing you've heard the saber-toothed tiger explanation? You know the one: Imagine it's thousands of years BC, and you have to run from a saber-toothed tiger—what happens? Your body turns on your sympathetic nervous system— your fight-or-flight hormonal stress response.

When that happens, without any conscious action on your part, your hypothalamus, located at the base of your brain, helps unleash a flurry of stress hormones and nerve signals that temporarily make your heart beat faster, widen your airways, and release stored glucose and fats to give you as much instant energy as possible. All of this is done for your benefit, so you're as fast and as strong as possible to either fight or run. But in order to do that, your body has to put a few things on the back burner, including your reproductive, digestive, and, most important, immune systems.

I'm sure you can see why this is a critical component of your body's natural survival mechanism. You are running from a f'ing tiger after all. And that's all well and good when you're dealing with potentially dangerous scenarios that require immediate physical action. However, once the threat is over, your body *should* flip your sympathetic nervous system off and turn your parasympathetic nervous system back on—your "rest and digest" or "feed and breed" mode, during which your blood pressure and hormone levels return to normal—or at least *should*.

Now, in these modern times, even though we're no longer running from tigers, stress has become omnipresent, creating a condition called chronic stress—and that sh*t is widely believed to accelerate aging[1] in multiple ways.

HOW STRESS AFFECTS YOUR AGE

When your stress-response system stays active, so does that steady stream of stress hormones, particularly adrenaline and cortisol. Adrenaline raises your heart rate and boosts your blood pressure for more energy, but left on, it inhibits digestion, affects your vision and hearing, and increases your risk of hypertension and stroke.

Constant cortisol is just as bad for your heart, but it ages you in ways that might surprise you. In addition to keeping your digestive and reproductive systems on the back burner, it affects the quality of your sleep, how well you remember things, and how well your immune system functions. That last one is a biggie, because that alone slows down the healing process and makes you far more susceptible to illnesses and conditions that ignite aging, such as oxidative stress, inhibition of DNA repair, and inflammation.

Nonstop stress can even reduce the effects of some therapeutics used to protect us from age-related issues. For example, researchers out of the University of Queensland found[2] that chronic stress in mice can have a debilitating effect on the immune system's response to cancer, reducing the effectiveness of immunotherapy treatments. This is why some experts believe that people with cancer should take medications that treat stress so that immunotherapy can be maximized.

Chronic stress may also recalibrate mitochondria structurally and functionally, particularly in the brain.[3] This is thought to cause widespread health effects, including an increased risk of disease and DNA damage that could lead to accelerated aging. Stress may even alter genetic activity, according to research[4] that discovered that some genes linked to stress disorders also affect our longevity.

But the consequence of stress that people find the most annoying is that middle-age muffin top, which comes out of nowhere and never seems to go away. And this is not from stress eating— which is a separate issue. Instead, it's that stress releases neuropeptide Y (NPY), a chemical that triggers the intra-abdominal fat cells to mature and fill up with more fat. To add insult to injury, chronic stress also stimulates a few genes related to inflammation and obesity. One of those genes, TBK1, has the power to turn off an enzyme that tells your cells to burn fat for energy. Without that enzyme churning, your cells burn way less fat—leaving you looking heavier and older.

There's even new data out of the Stanford University School

of Medicine that may help us understand on a molecular level why chronic stress causes weight gain. It might be related to glucocorticoids, hormones that do many things in our bodies, including suppress proteins to prevent inflammation and control how your cells utilize sugar and fat.

When you're healthy, your level of glucocorticoids goes up and down every twenty-four hours like clockwork, rising to its highest at about eight in the morning and triggering your appetite ("Rise and shine — now feed me!"). Levels then drop to their lowest at about 3:00 a.m.

But glucocorticoids also tell fat-progenitor cells to convert into adipose fatty tissue. Fat-progenitor cells renew and maintain healthy fat tissue. But they don't transform into fat cells until we need them to — and less than 1 percent actually transform if we're healthy. The problem is, your glucocorticoid levels are boosted by stress. And chronic stress . . . that can keep your glucocorticoid levels riding high all day long.

Scientists think that *when* stress raises those levels may explain why some people pack on more pounds than others. In a twenty-one-day study,[5] researchers gave mice pellets made with and without glucocorticoids. Even though they ate the same number of calories, the glucocorticoid group doubled their fat mass by both enlarging existing fat cells and — gulp — creating new ones! But when they boosted glucocorticoids by injection during the normal peak times of the day by as much as forty times, they never gained any fat. Like — nothing!

Could perfect timing be the answer for controlling stress weight gain? Maybe, say scientists, who now theorize that even if you get significantly stressed out, glucocorticoids shouldn't cause you to gain weight, just as long as whatever is stressing you out happens during the day. But if you experience chronic, continuous stress at night (sorry night shift workers!), it can create a change in your glucocorticoids that could both plump up existing fat cells and create new ones.

Even one bad day can affect how your body handles a cheat meal. Research out of Ohio State University[6] found that when women experience one or more stressful events in their day before eating a single high-fat meal, it actually slows down their metabolism. Yup, it turns out that stress combined with high-fat foods increased their insulin levels and reduced fat oxidation, causing stressed-out participants to burn 104 fewer calories during the seven hours after their meal compared to non-stressed participants.

Ready for something that will blow your mind? Even if for some strange reason, stress doesn't cause you to put on a single ounce, chronic stress can actually cause your gut microbiota (the microorganisms that are essential for digestive and metabolic health) to look exactly like the gut microbiota of someone who eats a high-fat diet—which is bad, BTW, and linked to a host of health issues.

Researchers at Brigham Young University[7] took a large group of mice and exposed half of the males and half of the females to a high-fat diet. After sixteen weeks of gorging, all of the mice were then exposed to mild stress for two and a half weeks. When they examined their gut microbiota before and after the stress was added, they discovered that among the mice that ate normally, the female mice (not the boys!) had the same exact negative changes in their bellies as those mice (male and female) that ate a high-fat diet. In other words, it took only eighteen days to achieve the same microbiota imbalance in their bellies as in the mice that ate a high-fat diet for close to four months. One of the study's authors suggests the gender discrepancy may be due to how males and females handle stress differently.

So what's the lesson? Don't hang out near saber-toothed tigers? Oh, wait, those are extinct. In fact, we're at the top of the food chain now. So, why are we still finding ourselves in fight-or-flight mode, and more important, why has stress become chronic for so many? This one is obvious, right? Or is it?

Modern life is still filled with stressful events. Some you can see coming…like having a new baby. Some are unexpected… like having your kid flush an entire roll of toilet paper, resulting in burst pipes and sewage-water raining through the first-floor ceiling. (Yes, that happened to me.) Most people think stress is caused only by things like these: the stack of bills piling up on your desk, relationship dynamics with your family or friends, or the long hours spent managing—or trying to manage—both of the above. Maybe you have two jobs and tackle a sixty-hour work week to make ends meet. Maybe you run around like a chicken with its head cut off shuttling kids from activity to activity, picking up dry cleaning, grocery shopping, and taking the dog to the vet. And at the end of these crazy-making days, you're left feeling depleted—like there is no room or time for your needs or the preservation of your sanity.

Now, it's highly likely you're managing one or more of the aforementioned scenarios. But the scary truth is, there are a variety of stressors beyond those, and it's likely your body is getting pounded by them from all sides on a regular basis.

Let's first look at what they are:

Physical: intense exercise, manual labor, lack of sleep, travel, long work hours, injuries or burns, surgery, illness, infections, extreme temperatures, extended exposure to UV rays, and so on
Chemical: drugs, alcohol, nicotine, and environmental pollutants and chemicals in poor-quality air and water; pesticides; cleaning products; beauty and hygiene products; and so forth
Nutritional: food allergies, chemicals in processed foods (fake fats, fake colors, preservatives, fake flavorings and sweeteners); vitamin and mineral deficiencies; nutrient deficiencies; dehydration; excessive calorie intake or extreme starvation, etc.
Psycho-Spiritual: troubled relationships, financial or career pressures, loss of a loved one, challenges with life goals, past childhood traumas, to cite a few

We all deal with much of the above at one point or another in our lives, and often the struggles seem to cascade and compound. You know, when you find yourself saying things like, "When it rains it pours," "I can't seem to catch my breath," or "I'm just waiting on those clouds to clear." Ever notice how the break never really comes? It only seems to get crazier with every passing year: a significant other, pets, kids, a mortgage, aging parents, more responsibility at work, possibly your own business, and so on.

So what do you do? Not live your life in order to avoid stress? Tell your parents they aren't allowed to get Alzheimer's? Not have kids? Demand a million-dollar paycheck so you don't need to worry about bills? Do you micromanage stuff so nothing can go wrong? Impossible. And it will only create more stress. (I know because I've tried.) You can't control everything. You're not God. No matter how many ways you play it, stress is inevitable because sh★t happens. In fact, the only thing you *can* control is how you respond when it does (more on this soon), and understanding, accepting, and capitalizing on this fact is what turns the tide in your favor. It allows you to not only mitigate the aging effects of stress but in many cases use stress to make yourself stronger.

Wait, what? *Stress can be good for us?* Heck, yeah! "We're stronger in the places we've been broken"—Hemingway, people. Need examples? No problem!

1. You work out for the first time in forever and you get blisters on your hands from lifting weights. In time, those blisters become calluses.
2. Your doctor tells you to lift weights for osteoporosis (porous bones). Weight lifting stresses our bones. Then bone cells migrate to the stressed area and begin the process of laying down new bone.
3. When you're out of shape, you get winded easily. Yet the more you run and the more you place stress on your cardiovascular system, the fitter you become—strengthening your heart muscle, increasing blood volume, creating new capillaries, widening existing capillaries, and so on, to pump and deliver blood to your muscle tissues.
4. Do you have allergies? I did as a kid. They were so bad that my parents opted to try immunotherapy in the form of allergy shots. That meant that I was exposed to the allergen in small amounts over time, which allowed my immune system to respond by producing antibodies to the dander, peanuts, pollen, dust, etc. Long story short...no more allergies for me.

I could go on, but let's dig deeper. Many of the stressful scenarios I referenced earlier aren't physical in origin. A divorce, while it has physical ramifications, is not a physical stressor. So how can those difficult, painful, sometimes frightening emotional and psychological stressors make you better or improve your life? The answer is in how you frame them.

If you can find your way into seeing them as life lessons, then healing comes in time. Great struggle and suffering can be transmuted into wisdom, depth, empathy, and strength—if that suffering has been given a meaning. And these lessons simultaneously grow your capacity for love, your resilience, and your ability to tolerate vulnerability and risk. Ultimately, anything in life worth having requires those three things.

I'm sure you've heard this quote about a million times: "What doesn't kill you makes you stronger." There's one caveat, of course. Handle any of the aforementioned examples wrong and you end up bitter, angry, and closed off, with torn up hands, broken bones, suffering from anaphylactic shock from a PB&J. Well, maybe not all at the same time, but you get the idea.

So what can you do to handle the stress? First, let's look at what's on the horizon.

WHAT THE FUTURE HOLDS

Science is hard at work looking for ways to combat chronic stress and premature aging by bringing the body back into balance. For example, one hormone, klotho, extends life span by regulating insulin and promoting better brain and body health. When it's lacking, it promotes aging by increasing your risk of atherosclerosis, decreased bone mineral density, and osteopenia. Recent studies have shown klotho levels are significantly lower in women under chronic stress.[8]

We're also getting closer to understanding how stress affects our immune system and its ability to defend us against disease, allergens, and other issues. A recent study[9] funded by the National Institutes of Health found that a specific stress receptor called corticotropin-releasing factor (or CRF1) actually sends signals to a particular type of white blood cell found inside bone marrow that directly interacts with bacteria and plays a huge part in protecting your body from pathogens. Researchers exposed two types of mice to different stressors—one type had normal levels of CRF1 and the other was CRF1-deficient. Those that had no CRF1 were better protected against stress. When exposed to allergic stress, they had a 54 percent reduction in disease, and when exposed to psychological stress, a 63 percent decrease in disease. The hope is that one day this know-how may help create therapies to treat the physiological immune-related effects of various kinds of environmental stresses. But for now, the best option for keeping CRF1 from screwing around with your immune cells is to try to control the stress in your life.

The most promising area of research is called "hormesis," and it focuses on the benefits of stress! Studies show that exposure to short-term, mild stress—both physiological and psychological— can actually have an anti-aging effect[10] by strengthening your cellular responses to stress. Theoretically, short-term stress promotes longevity by activating defensive molecular mechanisms and stimulating DNA repair. For example, Northwestern University bioscientists[11] have discovered that mildly stressing out the mitochondria in a breed of roundworm made the worms completely stress-resistant and doubled their life span. It also suppressed the accumulation of damaged proteins, which makes scientists wonder if controlled stress could help humans battle age-related diseases such as Alzheimer's, Huntington's, Parkinson's, and amyotrophic lateral sclerosis (ALS). There's even hope that one day we could use therapeutics to reprogram how our cells adapt to those stressors so they can better fight off diseases such as type-2 diabetes.

WHAT WE KNOW NOW

Turning the stress key in the right direction requires a holistic approach of eating right, exercising right, mitigating psychological stress, adapting your mindset to best manage stress's biochemical age inciters, and avoiding physical trauma and environmental chemicals as much as possible.

Again, while this may seem obvious, it isn't. And it isn't always easy. There are very specific ways all of the above must be handled, and what you may think of as eating right or exercising effectively could actually be counterproductive for managing stress. But don't worry—we will get to all that in part 3.

For now, here's a quick look at why and how these factors can best make stress work for you instead of against you, so when you do get to the nitty-gritty you'll know the methods behind my madness. Well, it's not really madness at all, but when I ask you to limit alcohol consumption, you might be a tad pissed. So, I'm priming the pump and giving you an incentive before I drop the hammer.

What to Eat

It's no secret that crap food raises cortisol, which is why sticking with high-quality sources of protein, low-glycemic and complex carbohydrates, and healthy fats can help lower your cortisol levels. Eating this way also boosts your immune system, keeps your blood sugar levels stabilized, and lowers blood pressure—all things that can get dangerously out of whack when stress is left unmanaged.

The catch-22: when you suffer from chronic stress, you're prone to increasing your intake of snack-type foods. We call them comfort foods, but there are several scientific reasons why you're reaching for crap. Studies[12] have shown that glucocorticoids (such as cortisol) trigger a need to eat foods high in sugar and fat.

Making matters worse, when you're stressed, your hypothalamus releases corticotropin-releasing hormone (CRH), which tells your body to release corticotropin, which in turn helps stimulate the secretion of corticosteroids (cortisone-like hormones). It's a vicious cycle: the more stressed you are, the more crap you eat, and the more crap you eat, the more cortisol gets released.

Alcohol consumption is another problem. A lot of people turn to alcohol as a way to de-stress, and there's plenty of research that shows light to moderate consumption actually seems to lower cortisol levels. One famous study[13] out of La Trobe University in Bendingo took a look at the effects of different types of drinks— white wine, red wine, light beer, and regular beer—on the hypothalamic-pituitary-adrenal (HPA) axis, which is responsible for the synthesis of cortisol. When participants ingested 40 grams of alcohol (about 1.5 ounces) four times, along with food, over the course of 135 minutes, they noticed that their levels of cortisol were significantly lower—the type of drink didn't seem to matter. However, severe intoxication (think binge drinking, or five or more drinks for men and four or more drinks for women in less than two hours) has been shown[14] to increase cortisol. Point being: having one to two drinks definitely lowers cortisol, but having too many can have the exact opposite effect.

We'll dig in much deeper when I explain the strategies that help turn the 6 Keys in the right direction. But for now, know that there are specific types of nutrients that inhibit cortisol production and nourish your adrenal gland so it can perform efficiently. And we will go over what to avoid so as not to exacerbate age inciters.

How to Sweat

If stress is so bad, then why exercise? I mean, that's technically stress, right? Well, actually, yeah. If you train too long, intensely, repetitively, or too often, the effects of fitness can be counterintuitive. Remember how I mentioned that stress from weight lifting could help you improve your bone density? Well, if you don't train properly, you could end up with a stress fracture instead.

Train wrong and you run the risk of taxing your system even more, injuring yourself, running your immune system down, breaking down muscle tissue, etc. Conversely, if you train the way I suggest, you will become fitter than ever. And yes, no matter how you train, your cortisol levels rise, but the effect is temporary and quickly returns back to normal. And training properly and consistently reduces your overall levels of cortisol and adrenaline. So just know that frequently stressing yourself out with a little exercise may cause a small, temporary spike in your body's stress hormones, but the benefit of exercise helps reduce those same stress hormones on a long-term basis.

How much exercise does the trick of reducing stress? Many experts point to exercising at least three times a week or putting in a twenty- to thirty-minute session each day. New data[15] has even shown that when you're under high levels of stress, doing some form of moderate-intensity activity for at least 150 minutes a week (five thirty-minute sessions) seems to be the ticket.

But how you work out to de-stress is really up for grabs. What you choose to do is entirely up to you. Sure, there's new data out on how running in particular may lessen the negative impact that chronic stress places on the hippocampus,[16] the part of your brain responsible for learning and memory. But that's true for a mouse—not a marathoner.

That said, taking time to breathe in addition to breaking a sweat can also turn back the years. Incorporating the kind of exercise that works as a mind-body intervention (MBI), such as meditation, yoga, and Tai Chi, doesn't simply relax you. MBIs can reverse the molecular reactions in your DNA that cause ill health and depression, according to a new study.[17] So by sprinkling in some mindfulness, you'll turn several keys at the same time. More on this one later, in chapter 12.

What to Watch For

This section on the stress key ultimately will be very extensive. As mentioned, there are so many types of stresses that we can suffer from and so many ways in which they must be addressed and managed.

Most kinds of physical, chemical, and nutritional stressors—such as injury; sleep deprivation; exposure to UV rays; chemicals in our air, water, or food; or vitamin and mineral deficiencies—can be significantly mitigated or avoided entirely with a little info and an action plan.

Even many of the psycho-spiritual stressors, including troubled relationships, career pressures, and past emotional trauma, can be managed, mitigated, prevented, and even transmuted into strength, wisdom, depth, and empathy . . . but you gotta bring the effort.

The good and bad news is that the list of to-dos is a bit extensive. Good because there is so much we can do and the impact can be tremendous. Bad because there is so much for us to address.

So this "what to look out for" piece is fairly extensive, and includes information on everything you would imagine can dramatically impact your ability to strong-arm chronic stress: sleep, socializing, sex, sunlight, meditation, psychotherapy—even organizing your life and your environment.

These are the habits, behaviors, and belief systems that can dramatically impact everything from your biochemistry to the physiology of your brain structure. Crazy, right? And we are gonna get into all of it—in great detail.

And this is where the real work begins. It won't be easy, and it will take time, but it will be worth it. I'll teach you how best to cope with worry, build support, bring meaning to loss, and reframe failures and setbacks so those hardships and stressors will make you stronger and work for you emotionally, psychologically, and physiologically as opposed to aging you and inviting disease.

The season that stresses you out the most!

If you live someplace notorious for its harsh, stressful winters, you might think that you probably have way more cortisol floating inside you when it's cold and nasty compared to when it's warmer outside. But some now speculate that the exact opposite is true, and that as the thermometer begins to rise, so do your levels of cortisol.

A new study[18] out of Poznan University of Medical Science in Poland looked at the circulating cortisol (and markers of inflammation) in female medical students during both the wintertime and summertime. Although their levels of inflammation never changed between seasons, their cortisol levels did rise in the summer. Why? It may have something to do with how the stress hormone also plays a role in adjusting the body's levels of salt and fluids—and how being dehydrated elevates cortisol as well. So even though summertime may feel more relaxing, keep in mind that it could be aging you in other ways than just more exposure to the sun.

CHAPTER 7

The Fourth Key: Owning Inflammation

First things first. Before I share why inflammation ages the hell out of us, and why managing it is a key to vitality, let's make one thing perfectly clear: inflammation is actually your ally. In fact, without it, you wouldn't even be able to survive the common cold.

Inflammation is your immune system's first responder, an ally that comes to the rescue to fight bacteria and viruses as well as to heal after injuries and infections. Your body manufactures certain immune cells and antibodies that attack foreign and bad-for-you substances, then certain hormones are released (such as histamine) that expand your blood vessels so all of those healing elements can flow directly into compromised tissue. It's that surge of extra blood flow that causes an area to become swollen, red, and hot. ·

Inflammation can even help your skin heal faster. Research[1] out of the Rockefeller University in New York City recently discovered that the stem cells deep within your skin responsible for replacing your skin's outermost layer actually remember how your body uses inflammation. That's right. Let's say you got a cut on your hand and it became inflamed. Well, the stem cells that helped patch up that cut have been found to form memories of that event. So the next time you get injured in the same place, your stem cells recognize the inflammation in the area and, as a result, respond even faster to heal your skin!

So what does this process have to do with aging? The inflammatory response is meant to be short-term. White blood cells go to the source of the problem; they start making substances that help other cells divide and grow to rebuild tissue and repair injury; and, once the immediate threat to your body is over, the entire inflammatory process stops. They call that *acute* inflammation, and it's entirely good for you. When it stays on active duty 24-7 (for a variety of reasons I'll explain in a second)—and inflammation becomes chronic—some serious age-related issues start adding up.

Are you noticing a theme yet?

As we age, there is a slow, gradual increase in inflammation inside many of us—a low-level form of inflammation that's both constant and destructive to our cells. It just doesn't turn off even though we're not injured or infected by anything.

What science now knows is that centenarians and others who have lived longer, healthier lives typically experience way less inflammation.[2] In fact, in a series of studies that involved 684 centenarians (people who were lucky enough to live to be 100 to 109 years old), researchers were surprised at how well inflammation predicted successful aging. When they looked at a variety of biological processes—including lipid and glucose metabolism, liver function, and renal function—guess what? Lower levels of inflammation proved to be the only consistent predictor of healthy aging.

It's *chronic* inflammation that keeps us looking and feeling older than we really are and makes us more susceptible to age-related diseases.[3] So how exactly is something that's meant to be helpful causing so much mayhem?

HOW INFLAMMATION AFFECTS YOUR AGE

When inflammation stays on, so does that flow of white blood cells and infection-fighting chemicals, all feverishly circulating around your body, battling a war that doesn't exist.

That may sound great in theory, but in reality, not so much. When white blood cells swoop in with no enemy in sight, they sometimes go after healthy organs, tissues, and cells. Instead of healing your body, chronic inflammation damages it over time, leading to issues such as rheumatoid arthritis, pulmonary disease, depression, and bone loss. It can also increase insulin resistance, raising your risk of diabetes and making it harder for you to lose weight.

And, your risk of cancer is also higher.[4] Over the last several decades, evidence has surfaced showing that chronic inflammation plays a critical role in tumorigenesis (the process of normal cells transforming into cancer cells) and that an inflammatory microenvironment is an essential part of all tumor formation. In addition, many other causes of cancer, like smoking, pollutants, dietary factors, and obesity, are associated with some form of chronic inflammation.

Chronic inflammation may even be why our skin ages[5] and why we lose muscle as we age — a culprit behind many age-related issues such as a slowing metabolism, higher risk of injury, and reduced quality of life. In a new study[6] out of Örebro University and University of Nottingham, researchers found that increased levels of an inflammation marker called C-reactive protein (CRP) seems to interfere with protein synthesis in muscle cells, which could explain the muscle loss. So if you're putting the work in and not seeing the results, it could be due to inflammation!

Another catastrophe chronic inflammation can cause is an imbalanced blood system. Within your bone marrow are blood-forming stem cells called hematopoietic stem cells (HSCs), which come to your rescue when you need to maintain healthy blood levels. The problem is that they are extremely sensitive to pro-inflammatory cytokines.

If you have chronic inflammation due to high levels of pro-inflammatory cytokines, it makes your HSCs jump into action to create myeloid cells (a type of immune system cell that fights pathogens) to help attack what they think is infection or injury. If those levels of "bad" cytokines stay high indefinitely because of chronic inflammation,[7] your HSCs never get a break from building myeloid cells. This then prevents them from regenerating and making other important blood and immune system cells.

So what's poking the bear?

Scientists feel that chronic inflammation can result from a number of issues, several of which are tied to macromolecular problems I mentioned in chapter 4. Our body can become less efficient at clearing out infected cells or folding proteins, so we rack up more damaged cells as a result. Having more damaged cells lying around keeps our immune system constantly on edge—so the inflammation switch stays on and begets an ongoing cycle.

Senescent cells also start to pile up as we age. Instead of dividing or dying, they sit around all day secreting pro-inflammatory cytokines. These molecules then affect the healthy cells around them, causing chronic tissue inflammation that can shorten life span and increase risk of cardiovascular disease and cancer.

And remember how I mentioned in chapter 4 that your cells can start sending the wrong messages to one another over time? That constant miscommunication can also increase systemic, chronic inflammation and has been linked to many age-related diseases, such as atherosclerosis and neurodegeneration. I'll say it again—it's all connected. In fact, a recent study[8] found that participants who had elevated biomarkers of inflammation in their blood in their 40s and 50s may have higher loss of brain cells decades later than people who don't, especially in areas of the brain linked to Alzheimer's disease.

Finally, it turns out that the inflammatory response activates a group of proteins responsible for controlling many genes involved in inflammation. This causes your hypothalamus to reduce how much gonadotropin-releasing hormone (GnRH)[9]—one of our primary anti-aging hormones—it produces, which can contribute to aging-related issues such as muscle weakness, fragile bones, skin atrophy, and decreased production of brain cells.[10]

WHAT THE FUTURE HOLDS

Here's where science is a little stuck: if you design a drug that shuts down inflammation, it leaves the body defenseless. Short-term inflammation is critical for cellular regeneration. Instead, researchers are exploring inflammation at the molecular level so they can develop drugs that specialize in "focused inflammation prevention." These treatments would only shut down chronic inflammation—not the short-term response that keeps us healthy.

In addition to strategies already being explored to remove

senescent cells (such as calorie restriction and senolytics) and restore specific macromolecules (like NMN and rapamycin, which seems to temporarily prevent senescent cells from triggering inflammation[11]), new strategies being considered to curb these overactive immune cells run the gamut from block-and-tackle to straight up outsmarting them.

One possibility is to reduce inflammation by blocking one of the molecules shown to contribute to it—interleukin-6 (IL-6). In trials, a promising new drug known as canakinumab, which can do just that, has been shown to decrease the rate of atherosclerosis by 25 percent and heart disease by 50 percent.[12]

Another is to trick immune cells[13] into believing they are running out of oxygen. You see, inflammation requires energy, and its main source of energy is oxygen. When a protein called hypoxia-inducible factor (HIF), a vital oxygen sensor in the body, is increased, your immune cells detect the extra HIF and think they're running out of oxygen. What do your immune cells do? They retreat, which in turn reduces inflammation. Scientists are hoping that this reaction may lead to therapies that may one day stop chronic inflammation by simply controlling this one protein.

But that's not the only one-stop solution being explored. What if you could trick the same hyperactive immune cells that cause inflammation to actually make their own biochemical that eliminates chronic inflammation altogether? That's what researchers[14] at the School of Biochemistry and Immunology at the Trinity Biomedical Sciences Institute at Trinity College in Dublin think may be possible after their discovery of a new metabolic process that appears to make macrophages, the cells in the immune system that cause inflammation, turn glucose into a biochemical called *itaconate*. Itaconate acts as a powerful anti-inflammatory, but so far, the process has only worked on mice and on human cells in a dish.

WHAT WE KNOW NOW

Turning down the dial on low-grade chronic inflammation requires tweaking some of the factors that are keeping your immune system in overdrive.

The good news is, by turning the First Key (Managing Macromolecules), you'll be minimizing free radicals and oxidative stress in your body, which[15] can contribute to chronic inflammation. But that doesn't mean there aren't other areas to consider to make sure you're not allowing inflammation to age you.

One of the biggest instigators of inflammation is obesity. The reason is that adipose tissue secretes adipokines,[16] pro-inflammatory cytokines that keep the fires lit. Reducing your body fat through diet and exercise, and eating as many anti-inflammatory foods as possible, can turn down some of that adipose-induced heat. Also, exposure to many of the things that screw around with your epigenetics can also turn your immune system against you. Be aware of environmental enemies that are good friends with inflammation, from the products you use to the air you breathe—all of which are outlined in chapter 15.

What to Eat

First, say no to a Western diet! Turns out that a diet high in fat, high in sugar, and low in fiber doesn't just make you out of shape—it turns your immune system into an aggressive beast. A recent study[17] on mice led by the University of Bonn discovered that unhealthy food makes the body's defenses hyperactive, and the inflammation it promotes can linger for at least four weeks after switching back to a healthy diet.

What's frightening is that it doesn't even take that long to create chronic inflammation by eating poorly. Scientists mimicked a typical unhealthy Western diet, high in sugar and fat, and low in fiber, and kept mice on it for a month. Almost immediately, their immune systems reacted as if they were fighting off a dangerous bacterial infection.

Staying away from pro-inflammatory fare is your best bet. Fried foods, too much dairy, too much red meat, processed meats, artificial sweeteners, refined sugar or refined flour products (such as white bread or pasta, pretzels, and many breakfast cereals, for example), and anything containing trans fats (such as baked goods, margarine, and many processed foods) can all cause systemic inflammation that accelerates aging.

Keeping your belly balanced can have a huge impact as well. Several studies have suggested that chronic inflammation is linked to imbalances in gut bacteria. For example, when gut bacteria from old mice were placed in the bellies of young, healthy mice, they experienced chronic inflammation.[18]

When "bad" bacteria become more dominant than "good" bacteria, your gut can become more permeable. Maybe you've heard the term leaky gut? This is it. It allows toxins to enter the bloodstream and wreak havoc, potentially resulting in inflammatory bowel disease, obesity, diabetes, cancer, and anxiety, to name a few. Why the elderly, in particular, have higher levels of bad gut flora is not fully understood, but researchers believe it is likely due to a combination of factors, such as reduced physical activity, changes in diet, and overuse of antibiotics.

Some scientists at Baylor College of Medicine and the

University of Texas Health Science Center at Houston even speculate that one day we might be able to slow down aging with supplements derived from gut bacteria[19]—but we're not there yet. For now, avoiding an unhealthy diet—one high in simple sugars and high in fat, saturated fats in particular—is a way to keep the scales balanced in your favor.

Keeping a close eye on antibiotics is another. Antibiotics should be used only when absolutely necessary, and only organic, antibiotic-free meat and dairy products should be consumed.

Conversely, consuming fermented foods like kefir and kimchi, which are high in probiotics (live beneficial bacteria), can help replenish your good gut flora. And eating foods with prebiotic (nondigestible) fiber, like apple skins and beans, helps to feed the good bacteria in your gut. The 6 Keys diet is rich in prebiotic and probiotic foods; you can expect all the details in chapter 13.

Studies show that the ideal diet for lowering chronic inflammation is high in fruits and vegetables (especially berries), cold-water fish, and whole grains, with moderate amounts of monounsaturated fats and omega-3 fatty acids through foods like wild salmon, olive oil, nuts and seeds, and avocados.[20]

According to the latest research,[21] adults who had a higher adherence to this type of diet were found to have lower levels of the pro-inflammatory C-reactive protein (CRP) and higher levels of adiponectin,[22] an anti-inflammatory cytokine that also helps reverse insulin resistance and may lower your risk of some cancers, and heart and liver disease.[23]

In addition, there may be an added anti-inflammatory advantage to eating so many vegetables and fruits, especially those rich in lutein, such as green, leafy vegetables, kiwis, grapes, spinach, zucchini, and various forms of squash. Researchers[24] at Linköping University in Sweden discovered that lutein seems to lower the pro-inflammatory cytokine IL-6. When they looked at the levels of inflammation in the blood of more than 190 patients, they found that levels of lutein synced up perfectly with levels of IL-6. The more lutein, the fewer pro-inflammatory IL-6 cytokines.

A diet that's rich in herbs and spices also has been shown to have anti-inflammatory benefits. Ingredients like ginger, rosemary, turmeric, oregano, cayenne, cloves, and nutmeg all have powerful natural anti-inflammatory compounds. Even light alcohol consumption offers[25] anti-inflammatory benefits. Could a few drinks a night that leave you light-headed help keep the brain inside that head younger and sharper? One classic study involving more than three thousand healthy men and women between the ages of seventy and seventy-nine found that having one to seven drinks per week actually lowered levels of both IL-6 and CRP. Recently, it's even been shown[26] that low levels of alcohol (up to a drink a day) may help the brain clear away toxins, including those connected with Alzheimer's disease.

Mice that were exposed to low levels of alcohol (which translated into about 2.5 drinks a day) experienced not only less inflammation in their brains, but also improved glymphatic systems. What's that? Think of it as the system responsible for giving your brain a bath. Your glymphatic system sort of cleans brain tissue by washing it with cerebral spinal fluid, helping to flush away waste, including the proteins connected with Alzheimer's disease and dementia (beta-amyloid and tau). In fact, studies have shown that low to moderate alcohol consumption is connected to a lower risk of dementia.

But go overboard and you will not only impair your gut and liver function but also bring on persistent systemic inflammation.[27] In addition, alcohol inhibits fat metabolism and can send estrogen levels soaring as well as potentially damage your DNA if overconsumed, hence the reason it's linked to various cancers like breast, liver, colon, and rectal cancer.

So, how much you drink is key. And the type of alcohol also matters. If you don't play favorites, then always choose darker forms of alcohol (red wine, dark beer, and even whiskey, for example) over light (gin, white wine, and light beer, etc.). Why? Because the harder the alcohol in question is to see through, the more polyphenols and other antioxidants it has.

But when I say "can't see through," I'm talking about the alcohol—not the mixer you may be pouring it into. The extra sugar in soda, juice, fruit, or other kinds of sweet mixers can contribute to systemic inflammation, so straight up is best.

Again, this doesn't give you license to Netflix and chill with a bottle of wine every night. There are strict guidelines around alcohol consumption that will be laid out in chapter 13.

Supplements can also help control unchecked inflammation. Yes, it's obviously better to get all of your nutrients from your food, but the reality is that our diets are simply not that varied. Trying to find, prepare, and eat many different foods becomes a chore, and the soil the food is grown in might have been over-farmed and depleted of nutrients. Or you might simply not like specific foods.

Like fish, for example. If you hate fish, consider taking a fish or krill oil supplement, which contains inflammation-fighting omega-3 fatty acids.[28] And that's not the only supplement you can bring to the fight. Here are a few to consider so you have an idea of what to expect in part 3.

- Antioxidants like vitamins C and E and alpha lipoic acid[29] have been proven to combat inflammatory damage because of their antioxidative effect and ability to remove free radicals in the body.

- Quercetin[30] is a flavonoid found in foods such as dill, buck-wheat, cacao powder, red onions, and spring onions. It inhibits histamine, which causes inflammation, and is both anticarcino-genic and antiviral.
- Spirulina is an algae antioxidant that reduces inflammation and boosts levels of the anti-inflammatory cytokine adiponectin.[31]

How to Sweat

Using exercise to drop a few unwanted pounds and reach your target weight is another powerful way to reduce inflammation. It's been proven[32] that higher levels of fitness are associated with having not just a smaller waist circumference but a lower degree of inflammation independent of body weight. It makes perfect sense, since the more fat you burn, the less adipose tissue you have inciting inflammation. Plus, it's been shown that losing weight can dramatically boost adiponectin,[33] helping to regulate glucose levels and burn body fat.

Exercise also triggers the release of interleukin-6 (IL-6) as an anti-inflammatory mytokine instead of a pro-inflammatory cyto-kine. That's right: the same protein that science is trying to reduce with the drug canakinumab is sort of a double agent. IL-6 generally raises inflammation when it's produced, but for some reason, when it's released in response to your muscles con-tracting, it actually switches sides and becomes a kind of cytokine that helps bring down inflammation instead of promote it.[34]

Research[35] has also shown that engaging in physical activity can significantly reduce levels of CRP in the body. It's when you train improperly, without acclimation to the intensity level, too hard and for too long, or don't allow for adequate recovery that you can sustain an injury, increase stress, and contribute to chronic inflammation.

For those of you who really don't like exercising, what if I told you that just twenty minutes a day could be life-changing for you? Literally. Just twenty minutes a day is all it takes to lower the chronic inflammation that could be aging you faster. New data out of the University of California–San Diego School of Medicine[36] found that just one twenty-minute moderate-intensity workout managed to activate the sympathetic nervous system, which suppressed the production of pro-inflammatory cytokines. When researchers had participants exercise on a treadmill at a pace that matched their fitness level (think moderate!), they experienced a 5 percent decrease in the number of immune cells that produced the cytokine TNF—a major pro-inflammatory protein.

So if less is good, what happens if you exercise too much? Researchers out of Monash University found[37] that extreme prolonged exercise (labeled as "more than four hours of exercise in one session," as well as "consecutive days of endurance exercise") causes the gut to allow intestinal bacteria (endotoxins) to leak into the bloodstream. This leakage can flip your immune system into high gear and trigger a sepsis-induced systematic inflammation response—but only if you're pushing yourself beyond your capabilities.

After examining the blood samples of athletes both before and after participating in a twenty-four-hour ultramarathon, it was found that people who overexerted themselves (particularly because they hadn't trained properly beforehand) had elevated endotoxins. However, those who were in shape and followed a steady training program leading up to the event didn't have the same response. In fact, they had higher levels of the anti-inflammatory interleukin-10, which kept their immune system in check and inflammation at bay.

What to Watch For

According to experts, a number of environmental factors may play a crucial part in keeping your body in a chronic pro-inflammatory state.

Let's start with the obvious: toxins, toxins, toxins. The same damn troublemakers that affect other keys: produce grown with pesticides, exposure to phthalates in beauty and hygiene products, bisphenol A in our plastic food containers, and heavy metals in drinking water (such as cadmium, aluminum, and lead) have all been directly linked to inflammation.[38] That also goes for any seafood potentially containing high levels of mercury, including mackerel, tuna, and swordfish.[39]

What you breathe can incite inflammation, too. It turns out that air pollution[40] from car exhaust, cigarette smoke (or smoke in general), mold, lead, benzene,[41] soot, dust,[42] and household products containing formaldehyde[43] is just as guilty of triggering widespread inflammation. So, in chapter 15, when we go over how to improve your air quality, pay close attention.

Finally, how you end your day affects your inflammation levels, too. Turns out that a good night's sleep greatly reduces chronic inflammation. In fact, not only are there dozens of studies that say so, there's even a massive meta-analysis study[44] that looked at seventy-two studies on sleep's impact on inflammation involving more than fifty thousand participants.

What was the consensus? Sleep disturbances definitely raise your blood levels of both interleukin-6 and C-reactive protein. Both of these markers are linked to chronic age-related issues, including heart problems, hypertension, and type-2 diabetes, which puts poor sleep in the same category as a bad diet and not exercising.

In fact, losing just a few hours of sleep has been shown to trigger a key cellular pathway that induces inflammation. When a research team[45] at the UCLA Cousins Center measured the levels of NF-κB (a protein complex responsible for controlling many genes involved with inflammation) in healthy adults who were forced to stay awake from 11 p.m. to 3 a.m., they were through the roof compared to levels in participants who were allowed a full night's rest.

But here's the kicker—more sleep does not necessarily mean less inflammation. Turns out that getting more than your fair share of sleep has the same effect[46] on both interleukin-6 and C-reactive protein! So what's the sleep sweet spot? According to science, it's seven to eight hours of uninterrupted sleep per night.

Sleep on it for their sake!

Getting at least seven hours of sleep a night lowers inflammation, and data[47] shows that it also protects against stress-related inflammation triggered by fighting with your partner.

A recent study found that couples who slept less had a greater inflammatory response to conflict the next day and higher levels of pro-inflammatory cytokines after discussing a marital problem, compared to couples who got at least seven hours of shut-eye. For every hour of sleep they lost, couples increased their levels of inflammatory markers a whopping 6 percent—a number that rose to 10 percent per hour if they argued in an unhealthy way. Even more reason to never go to bed angry—it ages you!

CHAPTER 8

The Fifth Key: Managing Metabolism

It's no secret that I've already written the book on metabolism—or have I? Well, I thought I had...until now. Don't get me wrong, my book *Master Your Metabolism* is not filled with bad or incorrect info—it's just incomplete. And this is because I looked at metabolism only as it relates to body weight and, subsequently, all the lifestyle diseases associated with obesity. I didn't look at how it is connected to aging.

Believe it or not, the ideal metabolism as it relates to age—and the ideal metabolism as it relates to body weight—can be in opposition. Let me guess: you think you're misunderstanding me, right? Isn't a slow metabolism the worst possible thing in the world? Well, I can tell you this: there is absolutely no question that a slower metabolism is linked to a longer life. Ever heard the saying "the candle that burns twice as bright burns half as long"? That's a pretty solid metaphor for metabolism. But don't panic if you have a fast metabolism—you can still live a very long and healthy life. The keys remain the same, no matter where you fall on the metabolism bell curve.

What is it about a faster metabolism that we think is so great? Just one thing: you can eat more and not gain weight, which ages you whether you gain weight or not because, hello, it causes oxidative stress. So that friend who could eat whatever she wanted and not gain weight, the one you wanted to punch in the face? Well, guess what? That's not so great for her overall health—despite her pant size.

And while obesity is unhealthy and linked to many life-threatening diseases, like cancer and heart disease, a slow metabolism doesn't make you fat—if you exercise regularly and aren't overeating. It really is that simple. I've actually had a slower metabolism my entire life and thought it was a curse until now. I had to be smart about my food choices and careful not to overeat, and I managed to keep myself perfectly healthy at 16 percent body fat (give or take). Now I am so thankful that I have a slow metabolism because it forced me to be mindful about what and how much I ate and, without intention, resulted in lowering my rate of oxidative stress.

Let's say you're the person with the fast metabolism, and you're thinking, "Oh my God, I'm screwed." Not so. There are a ton of things you can do to offset this oxidative stress, but before we get into that, let's discuss what metabolism is.

The faster your metabolism, the more calories you burn all day long, but how many calories you burn depends on a few things. You burn calories when you exercise—but you should know that already. You also burn calories during non-exercise-activity thermogenesis (pretty much any activity you're doing while you're awake that's not technically exercise). You're burning calories when you're at rest or asleep. And finally, you burn calories while digesting food—this is called the thermic effect of food, or TEF.

The thing is, when you metabolize food, it stresses your body. And when you overeat, you're creating even more stress. That's just one piece of the puzzle related to why overeating may lead to a shorter life span and a variety of age-related health issues, such as type-2 diabetes and cardiovascular disease.

But other scientists are looking at metabolism from the perspective of how the foods we eat get broken down. The reason? Because having certain nutrients either abundant or absent in our systems may inhibit or trigger autophagy, a process that occurs when your body needs to recycle damaged and worn-out cells for their nutrients, which in turn can reduce the risk of some of the age-related issues we experience.

No possibility is being left ignored, but does that mean that we shouldn't rev up our metabolisms to help burn fat? I mean, if having a slower metabolism may help extend your life span, is it worth doing things that actually slow down your metabolism, like not exercising, not sleeping properly, and not eating protein-rich foods (which require more energy to digest than carbs and fats)? No, of course not. Our goal is not to slow down your metabolism but to inhibit certain aspects of metabolism that accelerate aging and maximize aspects that help combat it.

HOW METABOLISM AFFECTS YOUR AGE

Your body spends every waking second circulating blood, eliminating waste, growing and repairing cells, controlling your body temperature and hormone levels, keeping your brain and nerves firing, breathing—you name it. And all these metabolic activities to keep you alive not only take energy—they take their toll.

The very job of keeping you alive creates metabolic stress, which over time results in damage to your cells. You can avoid some of it, but you can't stop all of it, because it only shuts off entirely when you shut off for good. And that is antithetical to our goal here.

But there's one other thing about your metabolism that changes with age—your body's ability to detect nutrients. Most people think the word *metabolism* only means one thing— how fast your body converts food into energy. But scientists understand that there are molecular events that relate to your metabolism—events that occur because of an ebb or flow of specific key nutrients that float about in your system as your metabolism does its job.

Your body is way smarter than it looks—right down to a cellular level. Your cells produce enzymes to process different nutrients (like glucose, for example), and they rely on a series of nutrient-sensing pathways to both recognize the nutrients and respond to them in the right way. Even though you have many nutrient sensors, there are four major nutrient-sensing pathways— insulin/IGF-1 signaling (IIS), mechanistic target of rapamycin (mTOR), AMP-activated protein kinase (AMPK), and sirtuins— that really matter when it comes to what ages you.

In a nutshell, it kinda works like this: your IIS (among other things) lets your cells know when glucose is present, while mTOR is specifically sensitive to amino acids (broken down from the protein you're eating) and lets your cells know when that's around. Then the two team up to signal when there's an abundance of these nutrients available. The mTOR and IIS levels rise in relation to how much you're eating and how often, and your cells are alerted to this smorgasbord of food. Once your cells notice that there's plenty of glucose and amino acids to go around, they spend less time seeking out damaged cells to break down for their nutrients. Instead, they start using all those extra nutrients to grow cells.

Eating too much as well as too often causes your mTOR and

IIS levels to stay elevated all the time, and the process of autophagy (the breaking down of damaged cells) shuts off. Your body figures, "Why get rid of damaged cells when I have plenty of nutrients and hormones floating around?" But the longer autophagy is off, the more damaged, misfolded protein cells start stacking up. This leads to protein aggregation, which can cause bad things to happen, including cell dysfunction and tissue damage that can eventually lead to disease.

The other two nutrient-sensing pathways—AMPK and sirtuins—work together as well, but in the exact opposite way. Instead of noticing when you're swimming in nutrients, they're more concerned with when you have fewer nutrients hanging around.

AMPK is the master regulator of cellular energy. In particular, it monitors levels of adenosine triphosphate (ATP), a chemical your cells both store and break down for the energy necessary to execute every biological reaction in your body. Once AMPK senses you're using up your ATP, it goes to work as a central regulator of both lipid (fat) and glucose (sugar) metabolism. The higher your energy demand, the more ATP you need, and the more your AMPK pathway is activated.

Sirtuins, on the other hand, look for high levels of nicotinamide adenine dinucleotide (NAD+), a metabolite that's present in every cell and helps facilitate DNA repair. When they see plenty of NAD+ present, sirtuins help adjust your metabolism and regulate many metabolic functions, including keeping your genome and mitochondria stable. But when there is less NAD+ to be found, something that naturally happens as we age, keeping those processes in working order isn't always your sirtuin's top priority.

Could a pill really help your sirtuins surge?

A trace nutrient known as nicotinamide riboside (a lesser-known form of vitamin B3) has been touted as an anti-aging supplement because it appears to elevate NAD+. But the all-natural supplement may also affect a few metabolic pathways—particularly sirtuins.

A recent study[1] out of the University of Colorado Boulder had two groups of healthy men and women between the ages of fifty-five and seventy-nine take a placebo or 500 milligrams of nicotinamide riboside twice daily for six weeks. Afterward, the supplement group experienced a 60 percent increase in NAD+, a boost that they believe may help activate additional sirtuins and promote healthy aging. As an added anti-aging bonus: those participants that started the study with stage 1 hypertension also noticed a ten-point drop in their blood pressure that translated to reducing the risk of a heart attack by 25 percent.

So, what's the bottom line when it comes to aging? Science is showing that higher levels of AMPK and sirtuins extend your life span.[2] The exact opposite is true of your IIS and mTOR pathways. When these pathways are activated and their levels are elevated, life span is reduced,[3] but when they're decreased—yup, guess what? There's an increase in life span. So the goal here is to get AMPK and sirtuins up while bringing IIS and mTOR down.

Why do scientists think these pathways affect life span? When AMPK is activated, it inhibits mTOR,[4] thereby increasing autophagy. Meanwhile, when some forms of sirtuins are activated (such as SIRT1 and SIRT3), they help heal mitochondria, improve fatty acid oxidation (so you burn more fat for fuel), and enhance the effectiveness of antioxidants.[5]

In addition, when these pathways get out of whack, oxidative damage and mitochondrial dysfunction are exacerbated, which screws with your nutrient-sensing pathways even more, causing your cells to lose their ability to accurately notice certain nutrients and effectively do their job. They call this deregulated nutrient sensing, and it messes up all those cellular processes I just referenced above, inviting disease and accelerating aging. It can also cause your brain to start sending signals for more food even though your body doesn't need it—your body just isn't recognizing the nutrients it's actually getting. Hence, more oxidative stress from more food consumption and excess calories, which only increases your risk of metabolic syndrome, obesity, and type-2 diabetes. To compound the situation, both obesity and diabetes can create chronic inflammation, which contributes to deregulated nutrient sensing. It's a cycle that we *must* prevent if possible, or at least interrupt and dramatically inhibit if it's already underway.

Ready for the interesting thing? As you get older, your IIS becomes naturally less active, which also lowers your metabolism.[6] I know, there's that slower metabolism again. I can't tell you how many women have come to me beside themselves because their metabolisms slowed after menopause.

And guess what?

This is actually a really good thing—if we tweak their diet and exercise regimen to fend off weight gain. Remember, a decreased level of IIS and a slower metabolic rate actually extends your life, and it's possible that this is your body's natural defense mechanism against cellular damage. Your body may know what to do to protect itself. You just need to work with it instead of against it!

WHAT THE FUTURE HOLDS

As we've discussed, studies show that when you restrict calories (generally by up to a third of what you have been regularly consuming), there's a damn near linear increase in life span.[7] And you already know CR affects several keys. But the key it may have the greatest effect on is your metabolism.

One of the first major studies to explore the metabolic effects of CR in healthy humans, the CALERIE (Comprehensive Assessment of the Long-term Effects of Reducing Intake of Energy) trial, recently found that reducing caloric intake really does slow aging, affect metabolism, and protect against age-related disease.

The study,[8] which involved fifty-three non-obese men and women between twenty-one and fifty years old, had participants reduce their daily caloric intake by 15 percent. Two years later, the participants lost close to twenty pounds on average, even though their basal metabolism slowed down. That's right—they actually lost weight, not with a revved-up metabolism, but with a slower metabolism, which is thought to prolong life. More important, participants also seemed to decrease systemic oxidative stress, and none suffered a single adverse effect from eating less, such as anemia, excessive bone loss, or menstrual disorders, in case you're wondering. This new evidence supports the hypothesis that organisms that eat fewer calories may experience the greatest longevity.

In response to what we know about the benefits of calorie restriction, researchers are studying compounds that affect the four most important nutrient-sensing pathways in the same way calorie restriction does—so, hypothetically, you wouldn't have to eat less to get the benefits of eating less. For example, metformin (a drug commonly used to treat type-2 diabetes) has been shown[9] to boost the activity of AMPK and influence life span in mice.

In addition, a lot of research is looking at two compounds that seem to impact your sirtuins and mTOR pathways in the same way as calorie restriction: resveratrol and rapamycin.

Resveratrol: This compound found naturally in grapes, red wine, blueberries, cranberries, and even nuts (such as pistachios and peanuts) seems to be a potent activator of sirtuins, particularly SIRT1. Resveratrol has recently been shown to trigger cell death (apoptosis) in human chondrosarcoma cells (a rare form of bone cancer) and significantly slow tumor growth.[10]

But that's not all: resveratrol has also been proven to preserve muscle fibers as we age, minimize osteoporosis, lessen the negative effects of a high-fat, high-calorie diet, and prevent age- and obesity-related declines in heart function in animal studies. Even just inhaling resveratrol seems[11] to slow aging-related degenerative changes in mouse lungs.

Rapamycin: This biological compound, produced by bacteria and first discovered in the soil on Easter Island (pretty cool, right?), has several clinical applications as an immunosuppressive (to help treat autoimmune diseases), an anti-proliferative (to help prevent the spreading of malignant cells), and an anti-tumor agent. But it also inhibits the mTOR pathway and has been shown[12] to extend the life span of mice.

There are more than a thousand clinical trials[13] either underway or completed on the effects of rapamycin on aging. The most recent to test the effectiveness of rapamycin in humans involved participants[14] between the ages of seventy and ninety-five given one milligram of rapamycin daily. After eight weeks, researchers looked for changes in metabolism, the immune system, and physical performance (measured by a handgrip strength test and timed walks).

Unfortunately, although slight changes were observed in things like red blood cell counts and hemoglobin—and it was determined that short-term rapamycin treatment can be used safely in older, healthy individuals—none of these results were clinically significant. However, we don't completely understand mTOR's role in regulating metabolism, and until we figure it out, perfecting any effective therapies to target age-related diseases in humans by manipulating mTOR is still a ways off.[15]

Researchers are also focused on NMN, which activates SIRT1 and promotes new blood vessel and muscle growth. When researchers[16] at MIT gave NMN to older mice for two months, their capillary density (the number of blood vessels responsible for delivering oxygen and nutrients throughout the body) was brought back to levels typically seen in younger mice—plus, it boosted their endurance by as much as 80 percent!

There's even work underway looking at glucosamine. You know it as the popular, naturally occurring chemical that treats arthritis and improves cartilage and joint issues. But did you know science believes it might improve your metabolism and slow down how you age?

One epidemiological study[17] involving more than seventy-seven thousand Washington State residents ages fifty to seventy-six showed that people who took glucosamine regularly significantly lowered their risk of death by cancer and respiratory diseases. In another study, when the supplement was fed to aging mice, it not only improved glucose metabolism (which helps protect against diabetes) but also increased[18] life span by close to

10 percent—that's roughly eight extra years if you're human. How exactly? It turns out glucosamine interferes with one of the enzymes used in converting glucose, so that your mitochondria use fat and amino acids for energy instead. In essence, it mimics a low-carb diet on a cellular level, even though you're not eating fewer carbohydrates.

WHAT WE KNOW NOW

Okay, even though we know metabolic stress is unavoidable— it's the side effect of living—that doesn't mean you can't manipulate your metabolism and dial down the damage.

What to Eat

Earlier I mentioned that one day we might be able to bring on the positive benefits of calorie restriction without actually restricting calories. But we can still get awesome longevity-boosting benefits today by simply not eating so damn much.

One recent study[19] had obese men and women rein in their daily calories by 25 percent for six days straight. The participants' macronutrient breakdown was 30 percent protein, 45 percent carbs, and 25 percent fat. After twelve weeks, the participants not only experienced a reduction in body weight of more than twenty-four pounds (on average) and a 12 percent decrease in arterial stiffness (a thickening of the arterial wall related to hypertension and high blood pressure) but also lowered their total oxidative stress by 25 percent. That's huge.

When you eat can also affect how much traffic your IIS pathway gets. In a recent study,[20] fit participants were placed on an intermittent fasting program, which is a diet that involves consuming calories at intervals (as opposed to throughout the day).

Subjects were asked to consume all of their daily calories in an eight-hour period each day for eight weeks—they had three meals a day, with 40 percent of their total calories at 1 p.m., 25 percent at 4 p.m., and the rest (35 percent) at 8 p.m. So they had a sixteen-hour period of fasting daily, they didn't restrict calories, and they did resistance training three days a week. After eight weeks, the participants had maintained their muscle mass, didn't experience any difference in muscular strength, and had decreased their overall body fat.

Avoiding sugary foods that stimulate your IIS pathway may also turn the time tide. According to data, eating large amounts of simple carbohydrates and dairy products that are high in sugar overstimulates your IIS pathway and has been associated with raising your risk of cancer and type-2 diabetes.[21] Keeping your blood sugar levels from spiking is another way to keep your IIS pathway less active. After all, the less sugar you have floating around, the less insulin your body needs to release in order to deal with it. Plus, high circulating levels of insulin have been shown to accelerate aging in other ways, from stimulating mTOR to contributing to progressive cognitive impairment and neurodegenerative processes. In other words, it makes your brain age faster!

This is why one of the keto diet's claims to fame is that it can help Alzheimer's patients, since it's an extremely low-carb (but high-fat) way of eating. Alzheimer's is now being called type-3 diabetes in some circles and is thought to be related to insulin resistance. Keeping those insulin levels in check is imperative for everything from your waistline to your brain health. Despite its current popularity, keto is *not* the way to go; we will discuss eating strategies in chapter 13.

Actually, I'll give you one reason right now that a ketogenic diet (throw in the paleo diet as well) isn't age-friendly: some versions of these diets tend to be too high in protein. Going overboard with protein has been shown to stimulate mTOR by bombarding your body with more amino acids that it needs. Since mTOR helps regulate protein synthesis, the more amino acids it sees, the longer it shuts down autophagy. Eating a moderate—not excessive—amount of protein is better for slower aging.

Finally, there are foods that boost NMN, which activates SIRT1, including broccoli, cabbage, cucumber, edamame, and avocado. Although human trials are underway,[22] there is evidence in mice that NMN is a great anti-ager and may be fast-acting. When a team from Washington University School of Medicine[23] dissolved NMN in water and gave it to mice, the compound appeared in their bloodstream within three minutes!

How to Sweat

Food may be key to keeping the Big Four pathways and metabolism in check, but exercise is definitely a huge component, too. Remember adenosine triphosphate (ATP), the chemical your cells store and use for energy? Well, when you exercise, you only have a finite amount of ATP inside your muscle cells, and it's not much—basically enough energy to last about three to four seconds. Then your muscle needs to get more ATP. In fact, your muscles have to continuously produce ATP if they want to keep contracting.

So how do they replace it? Once AMPK senses you're using up your ATP, it goes to work to help keep your muscles moving in several ways:

It produces and breaks down sugars. Once AMPK is activated in your hypothalamus, it triggers the production of glucose from the liver by reducing glycogen synthesis (glucose storage). It also encourages the breakdown of glucose into ATP.

It stops protein production. Protein production takes a lot of energy. But when you exercise, your body sort of freaks out and does whatever it has to do to conserve energy. AMPK brings that production down considerably so that you have more energy to spare.

It maximizes your oxygen levels. You need oxygen to produce ATP, and AMPK improves your oxygen levels by widening your blood vessels.

In conclusion, we want our AMPK pathway active because it's been shown to extend life span. Exercise is one of the most effective ways of making that happen, more specifically, high-intensity workouts and exercises that involve a lot of muscle contraction (multi-muscle movements through compound exercises) because these types of movements, and this type of training, require so much energy (and ATP) to pull off.

In a recent trial,[24] researchers asked two groups of healthy participants to cycle at the same speed for either thirty minutes continuously or in thirty one-minute bursts followed by one minute of rest (intermittently). They noticed that AMPK increased immediately after exercise—and metabolic fluctuations increased threefold—in the interval group, but exercising continuously didn't achieve the same effect. Ultimately, aerobic steady-state training doesn't activate AMPK pathways as much as interval training does. This is just one more reason why you'll see HIIT training in your exercise prescription. Lucky you.

But wait, there's more! Exercise also affects sirtuin levels. In one trial[25] involving rats of various ages, the animals either were kept sedentary or placed on a strict forty-minutes-a-day, twelve-week swimming regime. When the three months were over, those that exercised experienced improved function in both AMPK and sirtuin pathways across the board.

Not into swimming with rats? That's fine, because even though prolonged exercise (such as endurance/aerobic exercise) has been shown to increase sirtuins, you can pull off the same effect with resistance training—so long as you're working at a high intensity. In one groundbreaking study,[26] participants were exposed to six weeks of high-intensity interval training three times a week. Each day consisted of ten four-minute intervals with a two-minute rest in between each interval—for a total of sixty minutes. After six weeks, their SIRT1 increased!

There is even research[27] showing that performing low-load resistance exercise (using lighter weight that allows you to perform twenty-five to thirty-five repetitions per set, per exercise) as well as high-load resistance exercise (choosing a weight that allows you to do the traditional eight to twelve repetitions per set, per exercise) can stimulate your muscles to make more mitochondria (mitochondria biogenesis). Ultimately, exercise boosts mitochondria biogenesis, and the more mitochondria you have, the more sirtuins you have.

With that said, resistance training also activates your mTOR pathway. mTOR is often referred to as the main regulator of anabolism (muscle growth), so when you push your muscles using resistance training, you trigger protein metabolism and activate mTOR. Research[28] has shown that taking a whey protein supplement immediately after resistance training elevates mTOR even further.

So does that mean you shouldn't do any resistance training? No, because it's sort of a temporary trade-off. Yes, resistance training does activate mTOR—temporarily. But it also helps us to build lean muscle (among other things), preventing sarcopenia, the age-related decrease in lean muscle mass that can alter your activity level and drastically affect your quality of life. If you don't build and preserve muscle, you not only will look and feel older but also will increase your risk of age-related injuries. In other words, the anti-aging benefits that come from resistance training far outweigh the age-accelerating downside that comes from briefly boosting your mTOR.

When we boil it all down, the consensus is: Eat less. Move more. And drink red wine — you're welcome for this one.

What to Watch For

Ready for the good news? Diet and exercise remain the major game-changers when it comes to affecting your metabolism, so there are not many lifestyle choices beyond the two that can make a big difference. But there are a couple to consider.

How much sun you are exposed to — particularly ultraviolet B (UVB) radiation rays (the ones responsible for sunburn) — may influence your mTOR levels. Researchers looking into ways to reduce the risk of skin cancer by inhibiting mTOR have made a connection between UVB radiation and abnormal activation of mTOR, but the link between UVB radiation and mTOR signaling has not been fully established. Still, if you really need another reason to watch your sun exposure, there you go.

In addition, getting enough sleep seems to keep your sirtuin pathway humming. When a team of researchers[29] at the University of Pennsylvania School of Medicine altered the sleep patterns of mice to patterns ranging from normal rest, short wakefulness, and extended wakefulness (which mimics a shift worker's typical sleep pattern), they found that the levels of sirtuin type 3 (SIRT3) in mice that experienced extended wakefulness were reduced after just a few days even after being given time to catch up on sleep afterward. That means that even though you might "feel" fresh and fully recovered by repaying your sleep debt after a few nights of sleep deprivation, your metabolism may still suffer long after as a result.

Beyond that, it's all about food. It's all about exercise. With perhaps a little bit of effort also thrown at sleep—for now, at least.

CHAPTER 9

The Sixth Key: Tackling Telomeres

If you could look inside every single cell in your body, you would see twenty-three pairs of chromosomes (forty-six chromosomes in total). And at the end of every one of those squiggly little threadlike things are telomeres. These little caps on the tips of each chromosome protect your genetic information from being lost when your cells divide and keep the chromosome from fusing with neighboring chromosomes.

Think of them like the ends on your shoelaces, but they're not made of cheap plastic. They're made from a repeated series of DNA segments (or base pairs) repeated over and over again thousands of times. In white blood cells, for example, you start out with around eight thousand base pairs at the ends of your chromosomes. Over and over and over again, that base pair sequence repeats itself, almost as if you're winding masking tape around the ends of your chromosomes to keep them snug and protected.

But here's the catch.

When your cells divide, and they will about fifty to seventy times on average over their lifetimes, the ends of your chromosomes—well—they aren't copied quite as perfectly as you might think. Every time your DNA replicates itself and divides, it shaves a tiny bit (approximately twenty to thirty base pairs) off your telomeres. Oxidative stress messes with things as well and can cause you to lose an additional fifty to one hundred fifty base pairs per split.

Who cares, right? After all, a single chromosome has around 150 million base pairs. That's all well and good, but unfortunately it adds up, and over time causes those telomeres to shrink. And once a telomere becomes too short, it leaves your cell's DNA exposed. That's when a series of unwelcome biological actions can occur.

HOW TELOMERES AFFECT YOUR AGE

Size matters when it comes to your telomeres because if your chromosomes become too short they "lose their caps," so to speak, which can lead to several things. Your broken DNA might try to fix itself either by copying the sequence of another similar DNA molecule or by fusing together two cap-less chromosomes.

Neither is always a bad thing, and either can temporarily do the trick. But if two chromosomes fuse, the cell can also die or become genetically abnormal. In the latter case, your abnormal cells continue to divide and become potentially dangerous.

But that's not all. When the caps come off your chromosomes, your cells can no longer divide. Instead, they either commit cellular suicide (apoptosis) or become senescent cells—the same zombie cells I told you about in chapter 4 that can accumulate and wreak havoc.

That's why the shortening of telomeres has been associated with aging. As skin and pigment cells die, we start to see wrinkles and gray hair. Even worse, when our immune cells start to die off, our risk of heart disease, diabetes, cognitive decline, premature death, and a number of age-related issues increases.

Why do our telomeres get chewed up and spit out after every split?

Some believe that shrinkage is intentional and that telomeres work like a biological clock that lets cells know when their time is up. Others aren't so sure, since certain cells in our bodies actually produce telomerase, an enzyme that lengthens shortened telomeres, allowing a cell to reproduce indefinitely and make it virtually immortal!

Believe it or not, you actually owe pond scum for opening the door to our understanding of this enzyme, which may be able to help us live longer one day. That's right—that green gunk that floats on top of still water (the single-celled organism actually has a name: tetrahymena) is the closest thing we have to Wolverine. You can't kill the stuff!

When scientist Elizabeth Blackburn began looking at tetrahymena, she discovered not only that their cells never get old or die, but also that their telomeres never shorten. In fact, sometimes their telomeres grow longer. What she also noticed was that pond scum was wildly abundant in telomerase—and she earned a Nobel prize for this discovery (well deserved, I might add).

The problem? Most of our cells don't produce telomerase. There are only a lucky few that do—adult stem cells, embryonic stem cells, and, unfortunately, cancer cells. In fact, close to 90 percent of all cancer cells have telomerase, which is why they're so hard to kill.

I know what you're thinking. Just infuse yourself with telomerase and you should be able to lengthen the life span of your cells and organs, right? But that could come at a price, since all that excess telomerase could simultaneously raise your risk of developing certain cancers.

On the flip side, if cancer needs telomerase to flourish, then why not create anti-telomerase drugs to fight age-related cancer? Some cells—such as immune cells, blood cells, and cells within the ovaries and testes—use telomerase, so you'd run the risk of severely impacting wound healing, fertility, and your body's ability to fight infection. Clearly, it's complicated. So let's take a closer look at what can be done.

WHAT THE FUTURE HOLDS

What sucks is that if you suffered abuse, trauma, or cancer as a child, science says your telomeres will naturally be shorter as you grow up.

For example, one new study[1] involving 2,420 children from broken homes found that when a child loses their father, their telomeres are tweaked. By age nine, children who experienced such heartache through death, jail time, or parental breakup had telomeres that were, on average, 14 percent shorter. The death of a dad created the largest impact (16 percent), followed by incarceration (10 percent), and finally, separation or divorce, which shrunk telomeres by around 6 percent.

Even being a mom may influence your telomere length. According to new research,[2] women who have given birth to at least one kid have telomeres that are, on average, 4.2 percent shorter than those of women who never had kids. Mind you, a different study[3] discovered that having more kids reduced telomere shortening and could slow the pace of cellular aging. Which do I believe? Well, neither study factored in stress.

Which brings me to my point: you need to look at *all* the pieces of the puzzle at the same time. When I wrote my pregnancy book, I found studies that showed that a fetus's stem cells could rejuvenate mom—literally. In fact, if you're a mom, know that your baby's cells are inside you for decades after you give birth.[4] Therefore, my conclusion would be it's the stress of caring for children, not the act of having them, that shortens telomeres.

Many scientists still hope to figure out how to use telomerase safely to lengthen telomeres and turn back aging. Right now, telomerase is being tested as a way to reverse senescence in endothelial cells[5] (the cells that line your blood vessels), and the enzyme has managed to delay aging and increase longevity—without increasing cancer—in mice. But even though research into lengthening telomeres using telomerase is still in its early stages, that doesn't mean science hasn't been fielding alternatives to extend them.

Some are toying with using stem cells to lengthen telomeres. A group of scientists[6] has managed to create hyper-long telomeres in mice by extending them in vitro. After researchers manipulated their stem cells in vitro, the mice were born with telomeres that were twice the normal length—and they stayed that way (minus the normal shortening that occurs over time). But they also noticed that their cells racked up less DNA damage and were able to repair damage more efficiently, and the mice had a lower tumor rate.

Other scientists are developing RNA therapy—a procedure that inserts RNA directly into cells—to trigger the production of telomerase. However, it has only managed to lengthen the life span of cultured human muscle and skin cells, so that's only good news if you live in a petri dish.

Research into telomerase may help us finally understand why the liver is so incredible at regeneration but can stop functioning properly, leading to cirrhosis and liver cancer. A recent study[7] by researchers at the Stanford University School of Medicine looked at the liver cells (or hepatocytes) of mice and found that 3 to 5 percent of their hepatocytes seem to express abnormally high levels of telomerase—and these unique cells were also evenly distributed throughout the liver. As it turns out, these rare but well-placed cells seem to divide and form clones when either the liver was damaged or it was time to simply turn over new cells.

When researchers killed the telomerase-rich cells in mice, then exposed mice to a chemical that would damage the liver, they found that the mice that had no more telomerase-rich cells showed more severe liver scarring than those that still had them. Animal testing is so sh*tty, I know. So why do I bring that up? To illustrate that it could explain why the liver is so fast at repairing itself, no matter where the damage takes place. And if humans share this telomerase trait, then stopping cancer and cirrhosis in the liver may be as easy as protecting the few telomerase-producing cells scattered throughout the organ.

WHAT WE KNOW NOW

The good news is, by taking steps to improve the other five keys, you'll also protect your telomeres. For example, mastering your macromolecules by minimizing free radicals can help, since free radicals have been shown to speed up telomere shortening. Free radicals don't damage your telomeres directly; they damage the DNA that makes up telomeres as well as the DNA building blocks your cells use to extend them.

Lowering your stress level also has been found to be effective. Research suggests that cortisol and chronic stress, both cellular and psychological, can significantly reduce telomerase activation in immune cells[8] as well as shrink your telomeres. It's even been shown[9] that low-grade chronic inflammation can cause DNA damage in telomeres, so controlling inflammation could keep them nice and long.

It turns out that just a few smart lifestyle choices can fortify and even lengthen your telomeres. In one study,[10] participants switched to a diet high in fruits, vegetables, and unrefined grains; walked thirty minutes a day, six days a week; and practiced stress-busting techniques such as yoga and meditation. Over time, their telomeres grew by roughly 10 percent!

What to Eat

One of the most eye-opening studies showing the power of a Mediterranean-style diet on telomeres involved 217 elderly participants who were divided into three groups: those who did a half-ass job with the diet (low adherence), those who did a mid-level job (mid-adherence), and those who stuck to the diet as rigidly as possible (high-adherence). The stricter the participants were about sticking to a Mediterranean-style diet, the longer their telomeres were as a result.

Getting an abundance of nutrients — including magnesium and vitamins D, B6, and B12 — from foods such as fruit, vegetables, nuts, legumes, lean meats, and fish has been shown to protect your telomeres and keep those caps long and strong. And according to researchers[11] at Emory University School of Medicine, alpha lipoic acid (ALA) — found in spinach, tomatoes, and broccoli, for example — may stimulate telomerase (but so far, only in mice).

It's also been observed that foods high in beta carotene (think cantaloupe, sweet peppers, sweet potatoes, carrots, pumpkin, dark leafy greens, lettuce, winter squash, dried apricots, peas, broccoli, and even watermelon) could play a major role in helping telomeres maintain their length. A four-year analysis[12] of 3,660 participants age twenty years old and up showed that as participants' blood carotenoid levels increased, so did the length of their telomeres—by as much as 5 to 8 percent.

Even fatty acids are friends of your telomeres. Several studies[13] point to the protective powers of omega-3 fatty acids. Even better, research[14] out of Ohio State University found that adults who took omega-3 supplements for four months preserved telomere length in their white blood cells—the immune cells that fight off illness and disease.

What needs to be stripped from your diet? Well, for starters, since research has shown that a diet high in fiber and plenty of antioxidants is good for telomeres, it stands to reason that a diet high in empty foods (void of nutrients and fiber) is the exact opposite.

Staying away from foods that put you at a greater risk of obesity and insulin resistance—such as saturated and trans fats, fast foods, and simple carbohydrates like white rice and bread—is a smart move; both obesity and insulin resistance have been shown to shorten your telomeres.

You must throw out sugary sodas as well. In one of the first studies[15] ever to link sugar-sweetened beverage (SSB) consumption with telomere length (in a large, nationally representative sample of healthy adults), it was discovered that throwing back the wrong beverages could shave years off your telomeres. When the drinking habits and telomeres of more than fifty-three hundred adults between the ages of twenty and sixty-five (all of whom had no history of diabetes or cardiovascular disease) were studied, between 1999 and 2002, researchers found that daily consumption of twenty ounces of soda was linearly associated with shorter telomeres, roughly equivalent to 4.6 additional years of biological aging!

Impaired fasting glucose, increased oxidative stress, and systemic inflammation due to SSB consumption could all shorten telomeres. You can also give highly processed foods the boot. In one study of close to three thousand participants, researchers discovered[16] that for every daily serving of processed meat, the telomere length of the participants' white blood cells was reduced a teeny tiny bit! Surprisingly, when the researchers looked at unprocessed red meat, there was no reduction at all.

You may want to rethink one drink: coffee. One recent study[17] of nearly six thousand participants looked at the difference between caffeine consumption and coffee consumption. It was discovered that as caffeine intake increases, telomeres shorten. But the same investigation found that the more coffee you drink, the longer your telomeres tend to be!

For every one hundred milligrams of caffeine, telomeres were thirty-five to forty base pairs shorter. Conversely, for every one hundred grams of coffee (about 3.5 ounces), telomeres were found to be fifteen to eighteen base pairs longer. But who drinks 3.5 ounces of coffee, right? So think of it this way instead: for every cup of coffee (eight ounces), the participants' telomeres were thirty-four to forty base pairs longer. Is the answer decaf? Science hasn't figured that out yet, but since an average cup of coffee is about one hundred milligrams of caffeine, if you don't add sugar, it's sort of a telomere break-even.

So where does drinking alcohol fall into the mix? Scientists have looked[18] at the telomere lengths of four types of people: abstainers and former drinkers (zero drinks/week), low consumption drinkers (more than zero but fewer than seven drinks/

week), moderate drinkers (women consuming more than seven but fewer than ten drinks/week and men consuming more than seven but fewer than fifteen drinks/week) and high consumers (more than ten drinks/week for women and greater than fifteen drinks/week for men).

The consensus? Although scientists are still wrapping their minds around all the variables, it was found that even moderate drinking might not have a negative impact on telomere length. It doesn't extend them, but it doesn't really accelerate the shortening process, either. However, going overboard with booze too often could cause some problems for your telomeres. Research is now showing that both heavy alcohol use and binge drinking— consuming more than four drinks for women and more than five drinks for men in about two hours—can lead to premature telomere shortening.

How to Sweat

Regular exercise doesn't just build up your strength and endurance—it's preserving your telomeres. Researchers at Brigham Young University[19] recently discovered that adults who participated in regular physical activity (in this case, thirty to forty minutes of jogging five times a week) had telomeres that resembled those of individuals nine years younger who didn't exercise, and of individuals seven years younger who exercised occasionally.

Others have noticed that obesity may change how your telomeres age. When researchers[20] at the Medical University of Vienna in Vienna, Austria, looked at patients who experienced weight loss as a result of bariatric surgery, they found that their BMI (body mass index) dropped and they had longer telomeres up to two years later. The thought is that excess adipose tissue places the entire body under increased stress, which negatively impacts telomeres.

Even the length of time you spend either standing or sitting each day could be shaving away your caps in different ways. One study[21] involving a group of sixty-eight-year-old sedentary, overweight participants found a significant difference in those who sat more than they stood. The less they parked their butts, the longer the telomeres in their blood cells were after six months.

Recent studies seem to confirm that it's not only how long you exercise that's important but also how active you are when you're not working out. A landmark study[22] involving nearly fifteen hundred women ages sixty-four to ninety-five found that those participants who engaged in less than forty minutes of moderate to vigorous physical activity per day, and who remained sedentary for more than ten hours per day, had shorter telomeres. In fact, it was found that telomere length in the white blood cells of the most sedentary women was, on average, 170 base pairs shorter than telomere length in cells of the least sedentary women, which made them biologically older by eight years.

It's not all about intensity, though. Plenty of research is looking at meditation and other stress-relieving forms of activity that may have a positive effect on telomere maintenance. One of the most surprising studies[23] involved thirty-nine dementia caregivers (median age sixty) who were given two options: either practice Kirtan Kriya, a type of meditation with chanting involved, or listen to relaxing music for just twelve minutes a day for eight weeks. Those who chose music experienced a 3.7 percent improvement in telomerase activity—not bad, right? But those who opted to chant and meditate improved their telomerase activity by a whopping 43 percent.

But here's something both cool and confusing. So you know how resistance training builds muscle? Well, it doesn't really do much in terms of bulking up the telomeres in your muscle cells. But overtraining your muscles—through any form of exercise, whether strength training, too much cardio, or anything that leaves you in a state of not being able to recover properly—has been proven to shorten muscle-DNA telomeres significantly.[24] In fact, as it turns out, exercising too much may be just as bad for your telomeres as not bothering to exercise at all. According to research, there seems to be an inverted U relationship[25] between physical activity and telomere length—meaning, you sort of want to fall in the center of the U by doing moderate levels of physical activity.

So does that mean endurance exercise, such as marathon running, is out of the picture? One study[26] measured telomere length in runners before and after they ran seven marathons in seven days. Yeah, you heard that right—seven days! Despite all those steps, they found no change in the length of the runners' white-blood-cell and skeletal-muscle telomeres. This might be because the runners were already highly trained (so they probably weren't suffering from overtraining, in my opinion), or the amount of exercise wasn't sufficient to cause telomere shortening. Either way, the jury's still out on whether endurance training might negatively impact telomere length—but evidence sort of leans toward the positive.

Here's the deal: the thing to remember is that endurance training and overtraining are *not* the same thing. Sure, you may know a lot of people who run themselves (literally!) into the ground doing race after race after race. But done correctly—and by that, I mean allowing your body to recover properly—long-term endurance training may be very effective at lengthening your telomeres, especially as you get older.

In one study,[27] researchers studied two groups of male participants, one with a bunch of twenty- to twenty-seven-year-olds and the other with sixty-six- to seventy-seven-year-olds. In each group, half were endurance athletes and the other half exercised at a moderate level of activity at least twice a week. In the twenty-something group, there was no difference in telomere length in the two types of athletes. But in the older group, the endurance athletes (and these guys were all cross-country competitive skiers) had longer telomeres, offering some proof that endurance training—when done the right way—may allow your telomeres to go the distance as well.

What to Watch For

The first and most important thing to do is calm the f*ck down. And that's not me talking—that's science.

There's a lot of research to support that how you react to life events can impact your telomeres. One of the most comprehensive investigations[28] to date on the effects of short-term stress on telomeres—a meta-analysis that drew from every single study in all languages on the relationship between the two—found that the relationship between telomere length and perceived stress was approximately equal to the relationship between telomere length and obesity.

In layman's terms—worry and obesity cause the same amount of damage to your telomeres. Many scientists point to a classic study[29] that shows that caregivers of people with Alzheimer's disease are found to have significantly shortened telomeres. Experts believe that approaching any new struggle in life not as some massive, insurmountable threat but as a new challenge ready to be overcome might make a difference.

Current research also shows that conquering anxiety may help your telomere shrinkage problems. A study[30] of more than fifty-two hundred participants by researchers at Brigham and Women's Hospital in Boston, Massachusetts, revealed that a common form of anxiety (phobic anxiety, which 10 percent of the population experiences) was associated with shorter telomeres in women between the ages of forty-two and sixty-nine. The difference in telomere length was equivalent to six full years of aging!

Next up, depression delivers another blow to our telomeres — at least in birds. When scientists[31] at the University of Veterinary Medicine, Vienna, looked at the telomeres of African gray parrots kept in captivity and compared those that had a companion with those that were flying solo (so to speak) — the single birds had much shorter telomeres.

Although we don't yet have a lot of data confirming the same effect in people, studies on depression and white-blood-cell telomeres, as well as on depression and telomerase maintenance, are starting to show that depression does likely shrink your telomeres.

We've all been depressed at one point or another in our lives. Depression ranges from temporary, situational episodes of sadness to severe, chronic illness. And clinical depression (also known as major depression or major depressive disorder) is the most severe. Clinical depression isn't the same as depression caused by the loss of a loved one, or by a medical condition such as a thyroid disorder. None of these types, however, are great for your telomeres.

Usually, situational depression fades with time with the support of family and friends, counseling, exercise, and other acts of self-care. However, it can become chronic or clinical. If things compound, you must seek help, for a myriad of reasons that go beyond your telomeres. Consider seeing a psychiatrist to help you stabilize your brain chemistry.

The compounded effect of fear, anxiety, stress, and depression can be most damaging of all. According to research[32] out of the University of Pittsburgh, people who live in areas where there's a perceived sense of disorder, high rates of crime, and high levels of noise have significantly shorter telomeres than those who don't— a difference comparable to roughly twelve years in chronological age.

Here's one you will appreciate, I think: in a recent study[33] that examined the telomere length of 129 stressed-out mothers for just one week, women who reported sexual intimacy were found to have significantly longer telomeres in particular kinds of blood cells.

Sleep also matters, big-time. Shocker, I know. There seems to be a linear connection between sleep duration and the length of your white-blood-cell telomeres—at least in men. One study[34] showed that men who slept five hours or fewer nightly had telomeres that were 6 percent shorter compared to those of men who slept at least seven hours. Surprisingly, lack of sleep didn't have any effect on women. Still, new data might change all that.

Finally, we're just beginning to grasp how the air you breathe takes a turn at tearing up telomeres. If you smoke, you may be shrinking them[35] at a rate three times faster than nonsmokers. But what really sucks is that even if you don't, you're still at risk, especially if you live in an urban area.

When researchers[36] out of the University of California, Berkeley, looked at young kids living in Fresno, the second most polluted city in the United States, they found a strong connection between high levels of polycyclic aromatic hydrocarbon (or PAH, an air pollutant in car exhaust) and decreasing telomere length. Think that's bad? Scientists in China recently found[37] that babies exposed in the womb to high levels of PAH had shorter telomeres. That means that even before you're born, air pollution could be deciding how well you will age. Knowing that, you can see why it's never too early to start turning all 6 Keys in the right direction ASAP!

Teenage acne may help you live longer!

Did you suffer from bad acne as a teenager? Hey, that's great! Okay, well, maybe it wasn't *that* great back then. But as it turns out, acne sufferers' skin cells may be more resistant to aging. For many years, dermatologists have noticed that the skin of acne sufferers seems to age more slowly than the skin of those "lucky few" who didn't suffer from acne; the typical signs of aging, such as wrinkling and thinning skin, appear later in acne patients. This was always suspected to be due to increased sebum (oil) secretion. But recently, scientists[38] at King's College London found that people who have previously suffered from acne have longer telomeres in their white blood cells, suggesting that the delay in skin aging may be due to reduced senescence. In other words, your skin has fewer zombie cells now on account of all those zits back then!

Part 3

TURNING THE KEYS IN THE RIGHT DIRECTION

So...those are the 6 Keys. And I have to tell you that at this point in writing this book, even *I* have changed a few of my ways—in some areas, dramatically. And that's saying a lot because I thought I was crushing it when I decided to do this project. In fact, I was positive I was going to be my own poster child.

But throughout the process, with every sentence I wrote, I kept thinking, "Damn it! If only someone had told me all this when I was in my twenties. And if they did, if only I had been smart enough to listen." And again, I am doing amazing (if I do say so myself), but I honestly think I would have been that first person to live to two hundred, had I known at twenty what I know now.

It's not that I was wrong about things, since many of the age-changing details we now know about the 6 Keys are just emerging. But I was unquestionably functioning without all the pieces of the puzzle.

Now I understand the 6 Keys and how they affect aging, but that doesn't mean the hard part's over. I can't stress enough the importance of turning the keys in the right direction. Because how you eat, how you exercise, how you choose to live, even whom you choose to hang around—all of these things affect the 6 Keys and make or break which direction they turn. Follow the wrong strategies and your genetic potential will be locked away forever. But follow the right strategies and the locks holding you back from healthy aging will pop open.

If you're ready to see what's behind your door—then let's do this.

CHAPTER 10

Before We Begin

I must admit, when it comes to exercise and fitness, I have been breaking my arm patting myself on the back with each and every chapter. I can honestly say that my trainer logic—the way I put together my fitness programs and the techniques I use within them—is, and has always been, totally on point. If you are familiar with my fitness philosophies, the fitness component of the 6 Keys program will sound familiar—but it will be more detailed.

When it comes to lifestyle, I knew about the importance of greening your environment, managing your physical and emotional stress, and so on, but I didn't comprehend how diligent I truly needed to be on all these fronts. Sometimes I turned my air purifier on, but sometimes I didn't. Once in a while, I used beauty products that were toxin-free, but not all the time. On some days, I filtered my water, but on others, I drank it straight from the tap—blah, blah, blah. I don't want to make you feel like you have to be perfect, but the more you can make these age-resistant lifestyle choices a habit, the more they'll translate into years of life.

Now, with nutrition and overall diet, I'd say I knew about 75 percent of what there is to know about making healthy choices. That said, what's good for the weight management goose is not always good for the anti-aging gander, as we've discussed. Things like fasting, for instance: worst thing you can do if you want to be lean and to speed up your metabolism. However, fasting has tremendous benefits when it comes to anti-aging, if done properly. Alcohol is another big one: bad for weight loss but good (even up to two drinks a night!) for your heart health, cognitive function, and many aging-related issues.

Even the timing of when you take in your calories seems to make a difference. I have said for years that when it comes to your body weight, it doesn't really matter when you eat your food—all that matters is the amount of food you eat, as well as the quality of the food. If you skip a meal, you might overeat as a result. But if you ate a certain number of calories every hour for twenty-four hours or consumed all of those calories only once in twenty-four hours, your body weight would be the same.

When it comes to aging, though, the timing of your meals matters tremendously. If you constantly take in food, you throw off those nutrient-sensing pathways we discussed in chapter 8 (as well as a host of other things).

How about something like the keto diet? Yes, we know it can burn fat faster than other diets because it deprives your body of glucose and glycogen for fuel. However, keto is one of the absolute worst diets you can adopt when it comes to aging. There is no limit to the number of calories you can consume, so there's no possibility of achieving any of the benefits that can result from calorie restriction; and you don't eat carbohydrates, which are necessary for your cells to function properly. By default, on keto, you don't get many of the amazing antioxidants that fight aging (like resveratrol, for example) and you get too much fat (particularly saturated fat), which has been shown to shorten telomeres.

Finally, there are many studies that totally contradict each other when it comes to aging. For example, remember when I referenced a couple of studies on telomere length and having kids? One study[1] showed that women who gave birth had shorter telomeres by roughly 4 percent. Yet another study[2] found that in women who had multiple kids, the pace of telomere shortening and cellular aging slowed.

So why am I telling you this? Am I trying to confuse you? No. Am I trying to make you doubt everything you've just read? No. Am I trying to make you doubt all the advice I have ever given you? Absolutely not.

The bottom line is that I'm going to instruct you to do some things in this book that, more than likely, I instructed you *not* to do—or told you didn't really matter—in my previous books. And I'm about 99 percent sure that if you've ever read any diet books, it's entirely possible you've already encountered some contradictory advice. Note the aforementioned keto example.

The path I'm advising you to follow in this book is the most important one—above all others. And how do I know that? And how did I know whom to believe? Which findings did I embrace, and how did I marry the goals of being lean *and* living well past one hundred?

To answer that, we must first discuss how to interpret the majority of medical studies—and that's with a bit of healthy skepticism.

THE QUESTIONS TO CONSIDER

I have no doubt that you have likely felt the frustration of conflicting trends in science. One week, coffee is great for you, and the next it's the devil. The same goes with alcohol, meat, raw food, supplements, medications, and so on.

So what gives? Why can't we just come to a consensus on things? Or rather, why can't scientists? It's important to know the answers to the following questions:

1. *Who funded the study and why?* In the United States, many studies are funded by the government (such as the National Science Foundation or National Institutes of Health). However, many are also funded by private companies (for instance, "big food" or "big pharma" companies).

For example, a few years back, a study came out that measured the effectiveness of chocolate milk as a post-exercise recovery beverage for endurance sports. Who do you think funded the "chocolate milk is the most awesome post-workout drink ever" study? Wait for it . . . that's right! The National Dairy Council and the National Fluid Milk Processor Promotion Board. Shocker.

Similarly, physicians and medical researchers are paid large sums of money or offered stock shares to perform drug studies for pharmaceutical firms and food companies. Even the government can sometimes have its own agenda when it supports researchers with grants and other forms of funding because politicians take campaign contributions from big food and big pharma and then are indebted to those companies.

2. *Which factors were taken into account and, more important, which factors weren't—and why?* For example, in that telomere study relating to moms and how many kids they had, the researchers didn't factor in stress in any way. When there is a conflict in findings, one must look at all of the variables that could have influenced these different outcomes. As in, which stones were left unturned?

In many of those privately funded studies I just mentioned, the "why" is pretty obvious. A company might fund a study to back the safety and/or efficacy of its products. So the study might be skewed purposefully and the results cherry-picked to benefit the company. And, in some cases, although there may be no agenda, important elements might simply not be factored in or measured— they are just not taken into account (for example, the study on telomeres and having kids I just mentioned).

3. *Why would someone study the topic?* For example, why would a researcher think to study the effectiveness of chocolate milk on exercise recovery? How bizarre, right? Well, to get grant funding and tenure, and often just to keep the lights on, scientists and researchers have to get their work published in respected journals, where the majority of studies submitted are rejected. Unsurprisingly, many of the studies that tend to make the grade are those with eye-catching findings.

4. *What do your instincts tell you?* Honestly, at the end of the day, when I'm attempting to discern the truth, I listen to my gut. Meaning, if it sounds too good to be true, it probably is. If it sounds absurd, like chocolate milk being great after a workout, it probably is. And when all else fails, go beyond taking someone's word for it and look for other evidence, particularly studies that have been peer reviewed and/or replicated that show similar results.

I have spent years—literally decades—testing out so many different workouts and exercise techniques on myself and others I've trained. And ultimately, the results speak for themselves. I've seen with my own eyes what works and what doesn't. But it has taken patience, effort, and a thorough understanding of the subject matter—and that's exactly the approach I've taken with the 6 Keys.

In this book, there are hundreds of studies cited—studies that I have personally discussed with my tremendous cowriter, as well as with a host of health experts, including doctors, biochemists, registered dieticians, exercise physiologists, psychologists, and psychiatrists. And I have analyzed these studies in all the aforementioned ways. Each piece of information was reviewed from a myriad of angles—*without bias*.

The reason I have had so many *New York Times* bestsellers is that they deliver on their promise of credible info. Ergo, the truth has always served me because I serve it. And in my search for the truth on anti-aging, a theme emerged. One overwhelming, undeniable, powerful theme.

WALKING THE MIDDLE PATH

Have you ever marveled at starling murmuration, a phenomenon where literally thousands of starlings swoop with perfectly harmonized movements, twisting and turning in unison, making a massive flock of birds look as if they are one? (If you haven't seen this, I'm gonna need you to Google it really quick and then meet me back here.)

Okay, so you've seen it? Awesome. It's incredible, right? Bordering on magical? Scientists believe that the purpose of this hypnotic display is to help starlings defend against predators. But how in the hell are these birds so perfectly synchronized?

Well, this isn't an idle question. In fact, it's something that even physicists have been studying. The answer is pretty intricate, but ultimately, this marvel all comes down to balance.

These birds have an innate ability to perfectly balance individual effort with group cohesion to make their aerial ballet possible.

Now, I want you to think of all of the trillions of cells in your body and their unique responsibilities as starlings. When they work together in a harmonious way, your body finds balance and you can thrive for a super long time.

How do we achieve this balance? By respecting and maintaining the equilibrium of opposing forces, whether biological or psychological, within the body, the mind, and the world around us. We must avoid extremes, as they create imbalance, and always endeavor to walk the middle path.

What's so awful about the middle anyway?

The concept of "the middle" has taken on a negative connotation these days. The middle ground seems synonymous with compromise. The middle of the road has become synonymous with mediocrity. We have been encouraged to avoid this center.

In fact, while I haven't been around *that* long (forty-four years to be exact), it appears to me that as a society, we are the most polarized we've been in a very long time. We live in a culture that has, in large part, abandoned the concept of interdependence. We went from "it takes a village" to a rugged individualism that ultimately leaves us flying solo. We tend to associate extremism with religion or politics, but this bent toward extremes has infiltrated every aspect of our modern lives, from our pop culture to our ideas about healthy living. Let's step away from the big picture for a second and look at the trends over the last few decades in just fitness and nutrition. We have insane fitness races where people jump over fire, crawl under barbed wire, and perform extreme feats of endurance in extreme temperatures, for example, running through deserts for one-hundred-plus miles. One popular fitness craze had trainers with a weekend certification instruct non-Olympians to perform as many Olympic lifts as possible in a certain period of time. For those of you who don't know, Olympic lifts are intense exercises that require a lot of instruction and tremendous precision. And they were never intended, not even by Olympians, to be done according to time. Doing as many as you can as fast as you can? WTF? Who thought this was a good idea? And people got hurt, of course. Many of them.

As for nutrition, when you look at the fad diets over the years, nearly all of them advocate some form of extremism. You're expected to completely cut out fat, or animal protein, or carbs. Or how about the extreme fasting diets? The HCG diet, the 5/2 diet, the Master Cleanse, the juice cleanse, etc.? These diets promote extended periods of starvation. Five hundred calories? That's not calorie restriction; it's calorie deprivation, which damages healthy muscle tissue and throws off your endocrine system. I could go on and on and on.

Point being, health and longevity require a holistic, balanced approach. Everything is interconnected, and therefore an extreme approach to anything is destructive.

It's time to bring yourself back in balance

Think of the middle path as simply being centered.

When you think of the word *center*—what comes to mind? Here are just a few dictionary definitions:

As a noun:
- A point around which something rotates or revolves
- The source of an influence, action, or force

- An object balanced so that it is equidistant from all bordering or adjacent areas

As a verb:
- To come to a focus

What about the word *centered*? When you center yourself, you are literally *bringing yourself back to a place of balance* when life and all of its stressors try to knock you off course. Think about it. A centered person is one who is thoughtful and not impulsive. Reasonable and not irrational. Calm and not chaotic. Anchored and not unreliable.

Let me be a bit less theoretical for a second and show you how this concept manifests in your health practices:

- **Alcohol** is good for heart health, helps keep your liver primed, and has neuroprotective qualities. But drink too much (tip that balance) and it can damage your liver, contribute to breast cancer, and greatly inhibit fat metabolism.
- **Sunlight** is aptly named the sunshine vitamin because it's vital for our production of vitamin D, which helps our bodies absorb calcium, is essential for bone health, and has been shown to improve sleep, relieve stress, and help combat seasonal depression. Some research has even suggested that vitamin D might help protect us from certain cancers, such as breast and prostate, as well as heart disease. But, get too much sun and you have a host of problems, including wrinkles and skin aging as excess UV light damages collagen and elastic tissues in the skin. Take it a step further and you get skin cancer. Plus, that UV light also damages your retinas. Why do you think your eyesight goes at

forty? (I'm forty-plus and have worn sunglasses my whole life. My vision is still 20/20.)

• **Coffee** (particularly organic cold-brew coffee) can boost cognitive function, enhance athletic performance, and help to inhibit pancreatic cancer. It is high in antioxidants and can help type-2 diabetics by lowering blood sugar levels. However, if you drink more than four hundred milligrams of caffeine, you place yourself at risk for dehydration, insomnia, adrenal fatigue, and fibrocystic disease, to name a few potential problems.

I'm gonna keep hammering this with more examples to be damn sure you see the pattern:

• **Vitamins and minerals:** Just about every single vitamin and mineral is harmful in high doses; however, if you don't get enough of them, you're at risk of equally serious health issues. Vitamin C deficiency, for example, causes bruising, joint and muscle aches, dry skin, infection, and dental conditions, and if it gets bad enough, you can get scurvy for God's sake. At the same time, too much vitamin C can contribute to kidney disease and gastrointestinal issues. Some studies have even shown that too much vitamin C in supplement form can cause genetic damage and converts harmless ferric iron stored in the body to harmful ferrous iron, which damages the heart and other organs.

• **Calories:** This is an obvious one. Eat too much and you have obesity and all its related diseases (cancer, heart disease, diabetes, etc.). Don't eat enough and your body can stay in an extreme catabolic state where it's constantly breaking down tissue, a condition that can compromise your bone density, lean muscle tissue, immunity, and even your fertility. And nutrient deficiency begets a host of other issues.

- **Sleep:** If you don't get seven to eight hours a night, you run an increased risk of depression, a compromised immune system, obesity, cardiovascular disease, and accelerated aging. Conversely, sleeping *more than* nine hours a night can impair brain function, contribute to depression, and increase your risk of type-2 diabetes, angina, and coronary disease. Yikes!

I could go on...and on...and on. Because it's all like this. ALL of it. Every nutrient. Every habit. Every behavior.

Have you ever heard of the Goldilocks zone? It's the ideal distance that a planet must be from its sun to support life. Too close and you burn up. Too far away and you freeze. We have a biological Goldilocks zone, a zone in which the body is in balance and we are in ideal, prototypical health. Studies may show conflicting results, but if you take them all together, the answer is there, staring you right in the face: BALANCE!

Balance is not to be confused with symmetry or perfection. While something symmetrical can be balanced, ironically, balance in nature is often characterized by asymmetry.

In fact, you exist because of asymmetry. Let me explain. After the big bang, there was matter and antimatter, which annihilate each other. Fortunately, there was just a tiny bit more matter than antimatter—and that differential is one of the key factors that created our universe. I tell you this so you understand why perfection is not a tenet of this lifestyle.

Balance is not to be confused with moderation. While moderation in some cases may bring balance—for example, with alcohol consumption—moderation and balance are not one and the same. Balance involves give and take. Ebb and flow. It's a dynamic proposition that must be periodically reevaluated and tweaked.

Think of the teeter-totter you used as a kid. There you were, weighing in at about fifty-five pounds or so, and if a similar-sized kid was on the other end, you guys would happily and comfortably bounce up and down. But put that kid's dad on the other end and your ass is getting launched. Let your dad sit on your end, and once again, you have balance.

The point is, what may be moderation for someone else may not work for you. For example, an elite athlete's idea of moderation when it comes to exercise could be working out six days a week for sixty to ninety minutes because their body is already in prime shape. For you, that's probably way too much! Instead, it's about adjusting your habits and behaviors in a way that evens things out, according to where you are in your own life—and not someone else's.

Balance is not hard to find. You can find balance by observing how your actions affect your well-being, by acting on those observations when necessary, and, well, through common sense.

Crazy, I know.

This simple school of thought, while not always followed, *should* be obvious, no? We instinctively know how to care for ourselves. Our minds know and our bodies tell us. But we have gotten so far afield from what is our natural state that we have lost our way.

Not to worry. In the chapters that follow, I will take the guesswork out of this and give you a pretty exact formula to ensure you find your center.

In terms of common sense, let's clarify here and now: there is no room in your life for pesticides, trans fats, phthalates, parabens, BPA (bisphenol A), artificial colors, artificial flavors, high fructose corn syrup, or genetically engineered organisms. These aberrations are not naturally occurring and don't belong in our water, air, food, and hygiene products. They are some of the top offenders in throwing your endocrine system off balance and greatly contributing to disease and overall poor health.

I'll never forget the time I was asked to join a meeting with a high-level executive at a big food company. This woman tried to get me to stop bad-mouthing soda. She said: "Surely there is room for everything in a healthy lifestyle when consumed in moderation." I looked at the picture on her desk of her son and asked: "How much heroin do you think would be acceptable for your child to work into his healthy lifestyle?" Needless to say, we didn't end that meeting on super terms, and I have never and will never take money from big food companies.

So the path is clear. A balanced approach is the only way forward. It's the way we bring the 6 Keys into harmonious alignment for optimal health. Maybe you're thinking, *Balance? That's her big secret?* No. My secret is that there is no secret. There is only a universal truth. And always has been.

Yes, I will give you the exact formula to help you find your center. But that deeper theoretical principle of balance is the key to all the locks.

And maybe you're realizing I'm not the first to recognize this. And if so, you would be right. I'm not. In fact, it's something that we have known as human beings since the dawn of time. Yin and yang, equilibrium, and holism. The undeniable fact that everything is connected—including our 6 Keys.

These principles are reflected in nearly all the world's oldest healing systems, cultures, and religions. For example, both traditional Chinese medicine (TCM) and Ayurveda (Sanskrit for "science of life") are roughly three thousand years old and still practiced today. Both are complete systems of healing, encompassing aspects of biology, philosophy, psychology, and spirituality. Both assert that to be healthy, the forces within one's body need to be in balance—because where there is imbalance and disorder, there is illness.

A central tenet of indigenous cultures across the globe, from Native Americans and Aboriginals to African tribes and Pacific islanders, is that harmony and balance are the key to living a good life—free from sickness and conflict. And in these traditional cultures, harmony and balance need to exist in all spheres: in our physical health, our social health, our spiritual health, and our environmental health.

Even the majority of the world's religions espouse these same fundamental principles of oneness, connectedness, wholeness, and balance. Judaism, Islam, Christianity, Catholicism, Mormonism, Buddhism, Taoism, and Hinduism . . . each and every one gives a framework for how to properly care for your health. And their advice is extremely similar!

All refer to the body as a temple that needs to be clean both inside and out. All promote physical fitness and connect our mental health and physical health. All advise that food should be consumed in moderation, and nearly all recommend periods of fasting. All honor food with prayers of gratitude and have restrictions or guidelines of one type or another regarding meat (particularly the type and amount consumed and the way in which it is slaughtered). All recommend certain medicinal foods to optimize vitality and immunity, like garlic, holy basil, and pomegranate, to mention a few.

The path forward is undeniable. I want you to go into this with open eyes, an engaged mind, and a willing heart.

I want you to question.

I want you to study.

I want you to test.

I want you to tweak until you find your center.

And I promise you, if you search with sincerity, in the end, you will always find the truth.

CHAPTER 11

The 6 Keys Lifestyle Strategy

Surely you've heard the phrase "all roads lead home"? Well, the 6 Keys may unlock the door to healthy aging, but in order to open that door, you have to arrive at it first. To get there, you must travel along five paths—lifestyle, mind-body, food, fitness, and your environment—and all five are interconnected and converge at that door.

But while all five paths may lead to the same place, there is a necessary chronology to your journey. Before you can optimize your physical health and rejuvenate your body through diet, exercise, and looking at what's around you that may be aging you, you first have to center your mind. But before that's even possible, you must bring balance to your lifestyle.

When your life is chaotic, it creates stress and makes a calmer, quieter headspace significantly more difficult. Conversely, the more peaceful your life is, the more peaceful your frame of mind, and the better your physical well-being will be. It makes it so much easier to center your mind because the chaos is quelled. That's why we'll begin with lifestyle.

By the way, while the word *lifestyle* can apply to many things, from moral standards to socioeconomic brackets, for our purposes we're taking the word literally—the style of your life, or your habits and behaviors. Ultimately, if we can't change how we're actually living, then the other four pathways are inaccessible. So let's dive in.

The Twelve-Hour Rule

Now for the $64,000 question: how do you get your life under control so that each day is a step forward and not a step back? One word: *balance*. But you saw that one coming, right?

Let me guess: No time for self-care? No time for the gym? No time to smell the roses? No time to date? No time for friends? I've heard it all. You feel run ragged, spread thin, pulled in a million directions, and burnt out. I know you're struggling. But it doesn't *have* to be this way.

I have to make time for my kids, work, friends, physical health, fun, and so on . . . and there isn't one aspect of my life that's perfect—but my life is good enough. And your life can be good enough, too. So you're going to restructure it to make room for the actions you *must* take to help manage stress. You're going to allot a minimum of twelve hours a week to your well-being and physical health. That's the twelve-hour rule. I live by it, and it changed my life—dramatically.

You need this time. Without it, you can't achieve balance. Period. Don't tell me you can't, because the math speaks for itself: let's look at it.

If there are 168 hours in a week, and you spend 56 hours sleeping (8 hours a night), that leaves you with 112 waking hours over seven days. If you spend 50 hours on work, and you spend 50 hours on family and housekeeping stuff (laundry, taking the dog to the vet, doing homework with your kids, changing the oil in your car, etc.), that still leaves you with 12 hours.

Twelve pure hours of "you time" a week. Forty-eight hours a month.

Ideally, you'd be able to make even more time for yourself, but that is enough, and it makes all the difference in the world.

You could do the following weekly:

• Two to three hours of exercise (four to six intense thirty-minute sessions)
• Two to three hours dedicated to a date night
• Two to three hours spent on either a hobby or doing something with a friend
• Two hours of routine maintenance appointments (such as a haircut or doctor's or dentist's visit)
• Sixty to ninety minutes of meditation or any form of relaxation technique (broken down into ten to fifteen minutes a day)

You might rob an hour from Peter to pay Paul, but in general, it's fifty-six for sleep, 100 for your career and your home, and twelve for you.

To make the twelve-hour rule work for you, there's one thing you have to weed out entirely, and guess what that is? An extreme mindset of any kind on any topic. You must abandon perfection. Jettison the "all or nothing" mentality. Appreciate that you need help from others from time to time and don't always feel the need to go it alone. For example:

• Yes, a ninety-minute yoga class would be great, but the twenty-minute HIIT workout in your living room will work.
• Yes, it would be awesome to be parent of the year and go to every one of your kid's events. But honestly, making breakfast,

taking them to school, helping them with their homework, and having that bedtime heart-to-heart is enough.

• Yes, it would be awesome to do it all on your own and depend on no one. It would also be awesome to fly and be invisible, but that's not happening. You must be able to ask for help. Think of it as being on a team with family, coworkers, and friends. There is give and take. It's the only way. Remember, it takes a village.

• Yes, I get that kids have to come first, because they can't put themselves first, but that doesn't mean you have to be a martyr. It shouldn't be all or nothing; it doesn't set a good example for them of how they should manage their own self-care one day.

• Yes, I know you need a roof over your head and food on the table, but that doesn't mean that you have to answer emails at 9 p.m. on a Friday night or 3 p.m. on a Sunday afternoon.

Finding balance is tough at first. One of the biggest reasons we struggle with it is that it comes with inherent disappointment at the inability to be perfect. Or when we first realize that there may be things out of our control that make it much harder to bring things into balance. But you need to remember that's life. That people are not perfect. That you are not perfect. That they will disappoint you—and you will disappoint them. You can't control everything. Accepting the realities of life is hard, but the sooner you do, the sooner you can come to peace with them.

Balance Builders Beyond the Twelve

In addition to adopting the twelve-hour rule, there is a series of guidelines to follow that help manage the physiological and psychological stressors that can keep your life in a state of chaos. By adhering to these simple rules, you'll find yourself in a better place both physically and mentally to manage (and stick with) the other four paths I'll soon show you.

Sleep eight hours a night. No less than seven and no more than nine. This one is huge because as you now know, sleep affects every one of the 6 Keys. So make this a priority and do not cut corners.

Exercise two to three hours a week. This is such a major component that it has its own chapter. But in terms of bringing balance to your behaviors in particular, exercise reinforces the benefits and the importance of self-care and lends itself to deeper feelings of self-worth and self-confidence, hopefully making you feel that much more worthy of taking time out just for you. We also know that exercise enhances dopamine and serotonin (the feel-good brain chemicals), and that helps tremendously with managing stress — both emotional and physical.

Consider a pet. I'm a pet lover. It's no secret. I have about forty of them. Yes, I'm serious. A pig, four horses, three dogs, two cats, one rabbit, a parrot, fourteen chickens, four ducks, a wild goose, tons of fish, a desert tortoise, and a partridge in a pear tree (kidding on that one . . . sorta).

Have I gone overboard? Yes. I won't even try to defend it. However, study after study shows us that pets provide some pretty significant health benefits. Pet ownership can have a dramatic impact on infection control, cardiovascular disease, hypertension, cholesterol, allergies, stress, and psychological issues — all for the better. Much better, in fact.

Here are just a few of the findings.

• A pet can reduce your risk of a heart attack by 30 percent and your risk of a cardiovascular incident, like a stroke, by 40 percent.

• People with pets recovering from injury or surgery, or suffering from chronic pain conditions (for example, arthritis or migraines) require significantly less pain medication than those without pets.

• One study on children between the ages of five and seven found that kids with pets attended school three weeks more per year than kids without pets because they're sick less often and have fewer allergies (since pet dander acts as a natural immunotherapy to allergies).

• A Centers for Disease Control (CDC) study showed that pet owners have significantly lower cholesterol and triglyceride levels than those who don't own pets.

We don't know the exact reasons for all of the above, but we can make the safe assumption that some of it is related to the behavioral changes we make when owning a pet. Some animals intrinsically encourage a more active lifestyle and indirectly add exercise into your day. For example, dog owners have to walk their dogs and can add an hour or more of extra activity weekly from this alone.

Being a pet owner brings emotional and psychological benefits, too. The bond between people and their pets is significant, and most animals provide unconditional love, support, and companionship. This is good for not only our emotional well-being, but also our physical health. Our biochemical response to the affection we feel from our pets helps lower anxiety and stress.

That alone can significantly affect our body chemistry, enabling us to lower blood pressure and fight infection. Owning a pet also increases the release of serotonin to boost your mood, while simultaneously lowering cortisol levels, which helps control fat metabolism. Pets even encourage us to be more social—think about those trips to the dog park!

The conclusion is clear. Pets are great for our health. If you don't have one, consider getting one. I highly recommend rescue. There are literally millions of pets without loving homes. And I don't even wanna throw out the number of animals that are euthanized every year because they have nowhere to go. Consider saving a life, and I guarantee they will help save yours in return.

Meditate. For ten to fifteen minutes a day. I can't emphasize enough how significant this one is. And I had never done it—until writing this book. I thought of it like the cool-down part of a workout that most people tend to skip until they get injured. But study after study after study can't be wrong. So I downloaded some meditation apps and started working on it.

I've already explained that meditation can aid in stress management, improve the molecular reactions in your DNA that cause ill health and depression, and even help preserve your telomeres.

But I haven't yet mentioned that meditation literally changes your brain physiology and combats the deleterious effects of stress. Research has also shown that it may improve symptoms of stress-related conditions—including irritable bowel syndrome, post-traumatic stress disorder, and fibromyalgia[1]—and it helps relieve depression by lowering levels of inflammatory cytokines that are released in response to stress.[2]

Meditation also improves your immunity by boosting your antibodies. In a study[3] performed on biotech workers, participants who underwent weekly meditation training for eight weeks had significantly higher levels of antibodies than the control group. Another study out of UCLA found that when HIV-positive patients practiced mindfulness meditation, it helped them not only maintain but elevate their CD4 cell count (immune cells that typically drop when the virus is propagating).

Meditation has been shown to increase electrical activity in the prefrontal cortex, the right anterior insula, and the right hippocampus—all areas that control positive emotions and anxiety. These areas of the brain also act as a command center for your immune system.

And here is the super great part. Meditation is free and can be done anywhere. Start with five minutes a day, maybe first thing in the morning when you wake or at night before bed. You can even do it on your lunch hour in your office, car, or a park if need be. Build your way up to at least ten to fifteen minutes.

If you're curious what the optimal dose of meditation is, there really isn't a fixed answer because we're all different. We respond to meditation techniques differently and amounts of time differently. I recommend trying various apps, taking a class, or reading a book on meditation techniques to see what works best for you.

Minimize your sun exposure. Even though you need a healthy amount of vitamin D to keep the 6 Keys in order and stave off a variety of health issues, ranging from heart disease to breast and prostate cancer to osteoporosis, I don't recommend spending too much time in the direct sun.

What I do recommend is about fifteen to twenty minutes of off-peak sun time daily (any time before 10 a.m. or after 3 p.m.)

so that your body can produce enough vitamin D. Beyond that, whenever you're outdoors and exposed to the sun, cover up as much as possible and always wear a strong sunscreen that contains zinc (the safest sunscreen ingredient you can use).

Avoid any sunscreen that contains oxybenzone or retinal palmitate. Both are commonly found in sunscreen but have been linked to various health concerns. For example, oxybenzone is believed to interact with hormones, while retinal palmitate might produce free radicals.

Practice self-care. I'm talking about basic hygiene. And if you want to take it a step further with the occasional massage, facial, mani-pedi, and such, then have at it.

A study from the University of Miami's School of Medicine found that when participants were exposed to several weeks of massage therapy, their cortisol levels decreased, on average, by nearly one-third. In addition to keeping cortisol under control, regular massage also reduces stress by promoting production of those feel-good chemicals dopamine and serotonin.

No money for massage? That's okay, because even basic hygiene is extremely beneficial. Just the act of brushing your teeth and flossing (you non-flossers know who you are), conditioning your hair, filing your nails, and moisturizing your skin matters. Although these simple habits of routine body maintenance might seem insignificant, they can collectively have a huge impact.

Small acts of self-care maintain the health of your skin, soft tissue, hair, and nails (to name a few areas); keep you from getting sick; and help your emotional well-being, which in turn helps your physical health. When you give thought to and spend time on your appearance — not in a self-absorbed and unhealthy way, but in a caring and considerate way—you're reinforcing that *you* matter. It forces you to acknowledge your self-worth and recommit every day to your well-being, and this attitude benefits other aspects of your life.

Organize your life. This is definitely a personality thing. Some of us are naturally good at keeping sh★t in order and some aren't. Still, there is a way for everyone to find an organizing system that works for them. There's a reason the book *The Life-Changing Magic of Tidying Up* was a bestseller. Can you believe that? A whole book! Just on cleaning up and organizing your sh★t.

I have found that when my things are in chaos, it makes *me* feel chaotic. If I can't find a pair of shoes for a meeting, I feel rushed and scattered before my meeting. If my fridge is too messy and dirty, I feel so overwhelmed that I'll often just order in instead of making something healthy at home.

The bottom line is that you need to keep your environment free of clutter. Give everything a place and try to build in simple systems that allow you to easily access the things you need to function daily. Because when you don't have order in your life, it can stress you out mentally and, subsequently, physically. Plus, it ultimately wastes important resources like time and money.

Now, I am not an expert in this, but I am type A, so it comes pretty naturally to me. I recommend checking out that book I mentioned if it's tough for you to get organized. And, I *strongly* suggest you begin with a serious spring cleaning, even though it may not be spring. You need to make room for the new and give yourself some space—both literally and metaphorically.

Have sex. Yes, I know. Easier said than done in some cases. But if you don't have a willing partner, then take care of business yourself. Seriously. Get it done. Because ironically, when you're stressed, it kills your sex drive, and since sex is one of the things that mitigates stress — there's that vicious cycle.

The health benefits of sex are undeniable. It literally changes your brain and body chemistry and helps balance out hormones like estrogen, testosterone, and DHEA. It also releases a host of feel-good chemicals, including dopamine, serotonin, and oxytocin, which lower cortisol. One 2010 study even found that rodents who engaged in sex once a day for fourteen consecutive days actually grew more neurons in their hippocampus compared to rats who weren't as lucky.

Studies show that sex can improve immunity, lower blood pressure, improve memory, aid digestion, combat depression, lessen your risk of heart attack, and even help inhibit some forms of cancer.

Tough to argue with, right?

So how often should you be having orgasms? The research isn't conclusive, but it appears that once a week is the minimum to reap health benefits. Many studies I looked at on this topic appear to arrive at that conclusion. For example, a 2004 study from researchers at Wilkes University in Pennsylvania suggests that having sex once or twice per week leads to higher levels of the antibody immunoglobulin A. In other words, you're boosting your immune system by getting busy.

That said, get out there — or wherever you like to do it — and have more sex, because when it comes to aging, there is certainly no downside. Unless of course you have a sex addiction — which is a totally different conversation that's way outside the scope of this book.

Socialize. People need people.

Seems clichéd? Well, clichés exist for a reason. Like the other recommendations in this section, social support and companionship have been linked to everything from longer life and better physical health to improved mental well-being and a lower risk of dementia. I don't want to list a million studies because it will be the same exact type of stuff I listed before — but there's no escaping it. The research is out there; just look for proof in your own life. Getting love and support makes us feel important and less alone. It helps us cope with trauma and loss. It gives us meaning and a sense of belonging. Quality relationships make us happier, and when we're happier, we're healthier and live longer.

Here comes the part that reads like a cheesy self-help magazine — so forgive me. As stated earlier, each of these suggestions is worthy of its own book, but this is not a book about making friends. So here are the Cliffs Notes for how to expand your social circle and banish negative influences from your life.

If you have great relationships, make more time for them: Try to see your friends on a weekly or biweekly basis, minimum. Never take those relationships for granted or unintentionally allow yourselves to drift apart. Work them into your twelve hours, and if you can't find time to see each other in person, at least email, text, call, or FaceTime to stay in touch.

Think about building your base: Making new friends is equally important, but — and I speak from experience here — it's not always easy. I continue to put myself out there, and I'm happy to say I have about five great friends — lots of acquaintances, but five people who "ride or die."

Out of all the people I've met and tried to establish friendships with (and there have been many), five isn't much, but it's enough.

And having deep relationships with more people than that is tough to maintain anyway. This is a quality over quantity game. My point: be vulnerable, get yourself out there, and if someone doesn't respond to you, then their loss. For real. Fire enough bullets, and some are bound to hit the target. The ones that do are the ones that are meant to be.

If you're not sure how to make friends, try exploring community-based activities. It's a great way to find like-minded people. Try a faith community if you're religious. Volunteer. Extend and accept invitations. Attend community events. Take a fitness class . . . #fitfam. That didn't just come outta nowhere.

Take an inventory of your relationships: Conversely, if you have toxic relationships in your life, those are equally impactful on your health — for the worse and not the better. So if there are any toxic people in your life who drag you down — or make you feel less than you're really worth — end those relationships now. It is far better to be alone and take care of yourself than be abused or treated badly.

If there are people who don't respect you but you can't cut them out of your life — for example, a family member, your ex/ baby daddy or baby mama, or an unavoidable coworker — try to establish boundaries. Don't share things with them that they can make you feel bad about. Use intermediaries. Don't engage in topics that are charged if you can help it.

And if/when they disrespect you, don't allow it. Calmly say that you won't be treated that way, or blamed, or negated, or marginalized, and then walk away or hang up. Sometimes you have to teach people how to treat you, and the best way to earn respect is by respecting yourself. Be kind as often as you can — but take no sh*t. And don't lose your sh*t, either, if you can help it.

Because ultimately that's bad for your mental and physical health—and that means they win. F that.

Remember that less is more: Trust me—it's true. If you're older, you have probably figured this one out already. If you're under forty, well, it's likely you haven't. Between twenty and forty, we can spend our lives amassing things that only end up draining us and weighing us down. And between forty and sixty, we try to unwind and let go of all the crap we have entangled ourselves with.

Here's another cliché for you: "more money . . . more problems." I'm sure you're thinking, "Yeah, right. I'm worried about my rent [or my mortgage or my health care]."

I totally get that, but I believe that quote is about buying crap for all the wrong reasons, and then wasting your life managing or fixing all of it. Maybe you're trying to keep up appearances. Maybe you're doing it to please others. Maybe you're doing it because you think you should. Or maybe your ego is getting in the way. No matter what your reason, I guarantee that this will stress the hell out of you. Again, I speak from experience.

There was a point in my life when I had multiple homes, multiple cars, tons of pets (okay, that part hasn't changed), very young kids, tons of employees, younger siblings I had to care for financially, and aging parents I had to look after. I know . . . cry me a river, right? Well, if you're thinking that, then you're not wrong.

In large part, I was drowning in a mess of my own making. I felt like Atlas holding up the world—literally. I had a panic attack at forty. I had fallen into a depression and woke up one night thinking I was having a heart attack. My chest was tight. I was sweating. It was horrible. And that's when I knew things had to change. So I downsized big-time. I got rid of all the excess crap and simplified my life as much as possible. And it helped. A lot.

I appreciate that many of us have stress from the exact opposite problem—feeling like we don't have enough. In truth, this is the same piece of advice—less is more. There was a great study published in *Nature Human Behavior* about how much money bought happiness. The research showed that the number is really an income of roughly $95,000 a year. More than that didn't significantly bump up happiness—at all. The takeaway? You need enough to not stress about rent, but not so much that you are stressing about multiple rents. Get me? Cover your basic bases and stop trying to keep up with the Joneses.

Take it from me: more stuff equals more chaos, problems, and stress. But even worse, it means having significantly less time—and time is your most precious commodity. It really, truly is. I'm not saying you don't deserve nice things. I'm not saying don't build your career. However, too much is too much. And when you start spending all your time handling problems with those things or burning money to maintain those things, those things need to be rethought.

So here's our summary of action steps:

- Dedicate a minimum of twelve hours a week to your self-care and mental health.
- Sleep between seven and nine hours a night. No more and no less.
- Set aside at least two hours a week for exercise (either six twenty-minute sessions or four thirty-minute sessions).
- Consider becoming a pet owner if you aren't already.
- Meditate for at least ten minutes a day.
- Practice good hygiene and consider splurging on a massage from time to time.

• Clean house and keep your home, car, workspace, and any other environment in which you spend a significant amount of time clean and organized.

• Have sex with someone else or by yourself at least once a week.

• Socialize at least once a week with friends or spend time making new friends at community events.

• Get rid of the wrong people and the extra stuff. Less is more. Quality over quantity.

CHAPTER 12

The 6 Keys Mind-Body Strategy

We've discussed the mind–body connection throughout each of the 6 Keys. But in this chapter, I want to drive home how important your mental well-being is for your physical well-being, and vice versa. Knowing how to act on that information is crucial — and our action plan is fairly intensive.

Try not to be overwhelmed. Know that this part of your journey, above all others, will continue to evolve.

MIND-BODY BASICS

There are three critical points to remember:

1. What you believe affects your behaviors. Your behaviors dictate your actions — and our actions dictate our reality. To give one example, I can't tell you how many people have asked me to make "workouts for fifty-year-olds" or "seniors" or "menopause." But I don't. Why? Because fitness doesn't work that way. Your body doesn't say, "Oh, I've made 18,250 rotations around the sun. I can no longer jump, touch my toes, or lift weights." That's absurd. The difficulty and intensity level of your fitness routine is based upon your ability. And your ability has nothing to do with age—it has to do with how long you've been training and at what intensity. Period.

So if you've never exercised or haven't exercised in a long time, then you're a beginner—no matter your chronological age. If you have been exercising and you're quite fit, then you're either at an intermediate or advanced level, no matter your chronological age. However, if you think "Oh, I'm forty now and I need a workout for old people," then you stop training in the ways that keep you young.

We have mountains of proof on this. One Yale study[1] found that older adults with positive beliefs about old age are less likely to develop dementia, including those who are genetically disposed. The research also showed that exposing older individuals to negative age stereotypes exacerbates stress, whereas exposing them to positive age stereotypes can act as a buffer against stress.

Another landmark study by psychologist Ellen Langer in the early 1980s turned up equally stunning results. Langer followed eight men in their seventies over the course of five days in what she called a psychological intervention. Before the study, Langer assessed each man on such measures as dexterity, grip strength, flexibility, hearing and vision, memory, and cognition. Then she had all eight men move in together and told them to imagine that the clock had been set back twenty-two years. She surrounded them with memorabilia from that era and had them reminisce about when they were twenty-two years younger.

After just five days, the men were suppler, showed greater manual dexterity, and sat taller. Perhaps most improbably, their sight improved. Langer essentially put their minds in an earlier time and their bodies went along for the ride. How cool is that?

2. Your emotional state affects your biochemistry—and your biochemistry significantly impacts the 6 Keys. A quick couple of examples to jog your memory. Remember when we were discussing stress? When you're scared, worried, or anxious, your sympathetic nervous system (SNS) switches on and you release more adrenaline and cortisol, your blood pressure goes up, and your digestion, immune system, and sex drive get put on hold. Hence, the reason chronic stimulation of your SNS causes stomach problems, headaches, fatigue, muscle tension, sickness, cardiovascular disease, and so on.

Conversely, when you feel calm and centered, you activate your parasympathetic nervous system, which redirects your energy and biochemistry toward digestion and recovery, thereby combating the deleterious effects of age. So if you're chronically angry, jealous, guilty, stressed, depressed, or anxious, you're inciting a biochemical mutiny within your physiology.

As I mentioned in the lifestyle chapter, when we laugh, have fun, feel loved and supported, have orgasms (thank God this one is good for us), and stay in a positive emotional state, the release of natural opiates called endorphins—those super-duper feel-good chemicals (aka your body's natural narcotics)—is triggered. But these opiates aren't bad for you at all. In fact, they are great for you. They boost your immune system, relax muscles, elevate mood, and dampen pain.

3. What you think and feel can eventually become a physical reality. Our emotions and beliefs actually create physical changes in our brain structure and functioning! Floods of cortisol from stress, for instance, can shrink your hippocampus, which plays a key role in stress regulation and long-term memory. Meaning, being stressed affects your ability to handle more stress! The more of it you have in your life, the less effective you become at managing it.

It's either a vicious circle or virtuous cycle. If you're overcome with stress and sadness, it accelerates the aging of your brain and physically inclines you to be more stressed and sad. Conversely, if you can work gratitude, meaning, and mindfulness into your thought process, it can protect your brain and physically incline you to feel peaceful and more centered. So if you already veer toward the negative, we gotta change that. ASAP.

We used to believe that neuroplasticity, or the brain's ability to rewire itself, greatly diminished with age, but the good news is that current research has shown us this isn't at all true. We can recondition the way we think, respond, manage our emotions, and perceive the world at any point in our lives. When people say it's never too late to change, that applies to your brain's structure, cognitive functions, and aging process, too. You just have to do the work.

WHY IT'S IMPORTANT TO FIND PURPOSE

You've seen the evidence. What you think and feel matters when it comes to your health, youthfulness, and life span. Tremendously. You must make an effort to build more joy, love, fun, and other awesomeness into your life.

But even though I addressed some ways in the last chapter to build health- and happiness-making habits into your life, we both know that it isn't that simple. We can't be happy all of the time. Somehow, the notion that we can be, and that happiness should or could exist as a permanent state of being, has become mainstream.

There are literally hundreds if not thousands of books and podcasts meant to teach us how to be happy. And that pisses me off, because it's not real. That's not life and it only sets us up to fail and feel inadequate. Besides, if we were happy all the time, in my opinion, we would never learn or grow.

Of course I'm gonna tell you to make time for fun. Take your vacations. Follow your heart. Smell the roses. Seek joy in the little things. But here's the elephant in the room...what do you do when sh*t happens? And not just the daily annoyances like your car breaking down or your kid failing fifth grade. I mean those deep losses in life that can seem insurmountable.

How do we thrive despite all the sadness life inevitably throws at us—all the losses, failures, injustices, and tragedies? God knows we aren't gonna be happy about them. We can heal these wounds and become stronger in the places we're broken, and transmute these feelings into depth, wisdom, and empathy, but how? We do this by giving these losses, failures, injustices, and tragedies meaning, and by doing so, we find peace through purpose.

For example, I had a friend who lost her mother to breast cancer. After a tremendous amount of grieving she made the decision that the loss of her mom's life would be the thing that saved her life. She began exercise and eating healthy, and lost fifty pounds. She ran a 10k to raise money for a cancer charity and does so every year now. So you see, she gave the loss meaning and decided that something good would come out of something horribly sad. This is how you survive those types of losses.

WHAT'S YOUR *WHY*?

The necessity of meaning and purpose doesn't just apply to loss—it applies to EVERYTHING. Having an overall sense of purpose in life is crucial for longevity, happiness, and well-being.

And this has been proven. The evidence repeatedly shows that focusing on personal, meaningful goals can defend against the negative physiological effects of stress and anxiety.

For example, it's been found that people who have a higher sense of purpose in life are at lower risk of death and cardiovascular disease. Another study[2] that followed six thousand adults for fourteen years found that people who initially reported a strong purpose in life had a 15 percent lower risk of dying from any cause.

While further research is needed to determine exactly *how* purpose in life promotes health and combats disease, preliminary data suggests two mechanisms. One is that a sense of purpose provides people with motivation, vitality, and resilience to better handle their bodies' responses to stress. And two is that it gives them the sheer desire to stick around longer, and so it encourages them to live healthier.

Obviously our quest for the meaning of life is ages old in cultures world-wide. My favorite example is *ikigai,* a Japanese concept that translates to "reason for being." In France, it's referred to as *raison d'être.* In Native American culture, they have what they call vision quests. But in psychotherapy, it's called meaning-making.

Remember those two psychotherapeutic schools of thought I mentioned in the last chapter? Well, it's time to dig into the second one.

Meaning-making is how we become self-actualized and make sense of our life events and relationships. This process was first brought to light by Viktor Frankl, an Austrian neurologist and psychiatrist. He was also a Holocaust survivor. Sort of a hard left I just took there. However, it's the horrors that he experienced in the concentration camps that led him to discover the importance of finding meaning as a way to survive.

Frankl promoted the idea that meaning could be found even in the most unthinkable experiences of loss and tragedy. Although he didn't use the term "meaning-making" himself, his work influenced psychologists who later coined the term.

Frankl was inspired by Kierkegaard, Nietzsche, and Sartre, and in fact, used a quote from Nietzsche to set the tone of his book, *Man's Search for Meaning:* "He who has a why to live can bear with almost any how." In laymen's terms: if you have a meaningful goal or purpose, you can not only tolerate but actually grow stronger and smarter from the suffering, work, and sacrifice that is an inevitable part of life.

If you're at all familiar with my work, you know that I use this when working with people to create lasting motivation that enables them to stick to healthy eating and fitness for a lifetime. Now, I'm using this principle in a broader context.

When it comes to living longer and living well, what is your motivation to do so? What's your *why*? Do you even have one? And while the question is universal, the answer is unique. Here are just a few quotes by minds far greater than mine:

• "What matters is to find a purpose, to see what it really is that God wills that I shall do; the crucial thing is to find a truth which is truth for me, to find the idea for which I am willing to live and die. . . . I certainly do not deny that I still accept an imperative of knowledge and that through it men may be influenced, but then it must come alive in me, and this is what I now recognize as the most important of all." — Søren Kierkegaard

• "Meaning is not given and must be achieved. Meaning is something without representation or bearing in anything or anyone else. It is something truly unique to each person — separate, independent." — Sartre

- "For the vision of one man lends not its wings to another man. And even as each one of you stands alone in God's knowledge, so must each one of you be alone in his knowledge of God and in his understanding of the earth."—Kahlil Gibran, *The Prophet*

- "Ultimately, man should not ask what the meaning of his life is, but rather he must recognize that it is he who is asked."—Viktor Frankl

The point? That YOU must create meaning in your life and all that happens in it in order to truly thrive. Frankl outlined three ways to do so.

1. By creating a work or doing a deed. To me, this means identifying your passions and allowing them to be expressed, whether in your occupation or your daily hobbies and tasks. Aspire to your goals—and no one else's—and live for what you love, not for what you think you should love.

If you don't know yet what moves you, engage in a little self-exploration rather than simply observing what other people do. Think about your work history, education, hobbies, interests, and innate talents. Ask yourself what you enjoyed or found interesting, then cultivate those things by doing more of them. Be true to yourself. Find an outlet for your emotions and give them meaning through your actions. And finally, always try new things with an open mind and a willing heart.

2. By building upon your relationships. Cultivate a sense of belonging through your key relationships: your partner, your kids, your parents, your siblings, and your dear friends.

This is powerful. For some of us, it's the most important of all.

I know that even in my darkest moments, I would fight like hell to stay alive and well, even if just to be there for my kids, who have brought a new purpose into my life.

I'm not suggesting you allow someone to complete you or have them become your sole reason for living. But you can't argue with the fact that having love and support helps us tolerate the stresses of life, and the meaning in those critical relationships helps us to endure through even the worst tragedies.

3. By changing your attitude on unavoidable suffering.

Frankl didn't believe in being a martyr or suffering unnecessarily. However, he did acknowledge that in our lives, inevitably we'd be faced with hopeless situations and confronted with fates that can't be changed. He also knew that what can never be taken from us is how we choose to respond, and that bringing meaning to these difficult situations is truly the only way forward.

I can personally tell you that once I realized there was no such thing as smooth sailing in life, I learned to find peace in the calm before the storm, or in the eye of the storm, or in between the swells, where I can regroup, learn, grow stronger, and restore myself before getting pummeled again. My point is you need to find peace of mind, joy, and calm wherever and whenever you can. No matter how fleeting. Because it all matters.

I remember lying in bed one night during a particularly difficult period in my life, and instead of feeling dread for what the next day would bring, I just thought, *In this moment, I'm in my comfortable bed.* I relished in the physical feeling of my soft sheets and told myself, *I have at least eight hours before something can come at me again, and for this period, I have peace, quiet, and comfort.* Use these moments, no matter how brief, because they build resilience and help calm stress and anxiety.

Gratitude is another important factor in finding purpose. It reminds us of why life is good and how blessed we are to have time on this planet to experience all the incredible things the world has to offer us.

I used to have huge issues with the word *gratitude*. Phrases like "I'm so grateful I have my health" often made me think, *But what about the people who don't?* And that would always get me thinking about how unfair life can be.

I also felt like I had worked hard for what I had in my life, so why feel gratitude if I had earned those things myself? God I was stupid. I have since learned that gratitude means enjoying the good moments—period. When you feel good physically, you must allow yourself to be truly present in that moment and enjoy it. When you are in love, you must do the same. And when you eat something delicious, you should take your time to enjoy it. Being grateful is about pausing to be present so that you truly experience life in all its wonder.

I know what you're thinking. That maybe certain horrible things in life can't be reasoned with or rationalized, and no amount of gratitude or meaning can overcome them—but that isn't so. In fact, you must find meaning, just as Frankl did in the concentration camps after losing his life's work and almost his entire family, and experiencing tremendous suffering, both emotionally and physically. Yes, this is a hideous example, but the point is that if he could do it, then so can you. And out of that tragedy, he created logotherapy, a form of therapy meant to help others overcome tragedy as well. So much beauty is born from sadness and loss, including great works of art, books, ideas, and in Frankl's case, philosophies.

You *can* find meaning in trauma and tragedy, and in fact, your sanity and health depend on it. In my book *Unlimited,* I posed a question that I still find equally relevant today, and that's this: how can the evils or tragedies that may have befallen you provide an entry point for goodness on this planet? This is a HUGE question — I can't answer it for you. You'll have to take it with you and answer it as you go about the work of life. YOU are the one who must bring the meaning. All I can do is tell you it's there if you look for it. The application of this philosophy isn't easy. No true victory ever is. But we are programmed survivors, and you can get through ANYTHING if you lean into it, learn from it, and transform it.

Ultimately, you can derive inspiration and create purpose from many aspects of your life: religion or spirituality, work, relationships, and even loss. But the bottom line is that leading by your heart, feeding your passions, finding your meaning, and following your purpose are essential to a long, healthy, and fulfilling life.

So here's our summary of action steps:

- Remember that what you believe affects your behaviors.
- Remember that your emotional state affects your biochemistry and can significantly impact the 6 Keys.
- Remember that what you think and feel can eventually become a physical reality.
- Find your purpose in life — find your *why*.
- Continuously try to create a work or do a deed that's tied into your passions and allows them to be expressed.
    ○ Aspire to your goals — and no one else's — and live for what you love, not for what you think you should love.
    ○ If you don't know what moves you, think about your work history, education, hobbies, interests, and innate

talents; ask yourself what you enjoy or find interesting; then cultivate those things by doing more of them.

  ○ Always try new things with an open mind and a willing heart.

- Build upon all of your key relationships (your partner, kids, parents, siblings, and dear friends).
- Change your attitude about unavoidable suffering and find meaning in it.
- Be grateful and find purpose in everything—even the most tragic things in life.

CHAPTER 13

The 6 Keys Eating Strategy

Before there was keto, paleo, Atkins, gluten-free, fat-free, blood-type, HCG, 5/2, and so on — there was the balanced diet. A simple concept based on a simple, self-evident truth.

This should be obvious and speak for itself. Unfortunately, the world of proper nutrition has become so clouded by charlatans, snake-oil salesmen, and BS that most of us don't even know what a balanced diet looks like anymore. Not to worry, because we have an entire chapter to lay it out and if that isn't enough, I've even built a 6 Keys meal plan complete with hundreds of recipes into the Jillian Michaels My Fitness App if you want to go the extra mile. You can check it out here: https://www.jillian michaels.com/6keys2app.

CALORIES

A calorie is a unit of energy, and for our purposes it refers to a unit of energy in your food. But it goes far beyond being fit or being fat. It's about longevity, too. And while being overweight does have a significant negative impact on the 6 Keys, the nutrients in your calories, and the oxidative stress caused by eating too many calories, are also incredibly important.

So, calories matter—a lot. How many you eat. When you eat them. And the quality of the calories you eat. So let's break down each of these three.

HOW MUCH SHOULD YOU EAT?

We have tossed around the term calorie restriction (CR) dozens of times in the 6 Keys chapters. But before I can work CR into your life, we need to determine two things: your active metabolic rate (AMR) and its relationship to your health and fitness goals.

Your AMR is a combination of your basal metabolic rate (or BMR—the amount of energy your body uses in a day just for involuntary bodily functions like breathing, cell division, growing hair, etc.) and the energy you burn through activity, which includes exercise.

Now, if you wear a device (like an Apple watch) that tracks your calories burned, fantastic. If you don't, here's how you get a relatively accurate determination of what your AMR is.

1. Calculate your BMR. The BMR formula uses the variables of height, weight, age, and gender to calculate your body's energy expenditure. The only factors it leaves out are lean body mass (the ratio of muscle to fat) and biochemistry. For example, if you have hypothyroidism, PCOS, insulin resistance, estrogen dominance—there is no way for the BMR formula to reflect that. (You need blood work and an endocrinologist to determine your BMR when dealing with these issues.) But barring a hormonal disorder, this equation is fairly accurate.

One additional caveat: if you're very muscular, the calorie

burn will be slightly underestimated. And if you have a higher percentage of body fat, it will be slightly overestimated.

Use the following formula to calculate your BMR:

- **Women:** BMR = 655 + (4.35 x weight in pounds) + (4.7 x height in inches) − (4.7 x age in years)
- **Men:** BMR = 66 + (6.23 x weight in pounds) + (12.7 x height in inches) − (6.8 x age in years)

2. Figure out your daily activity score. Once you have your BMR, you need to think about how active you are during an average day. Identify which of the following most describes you:

- If you're chained to your desk and sedentary most of your day, you're a 1.1. People who fall into this category would be receptionists, telemarketers, customer service reps, etc.
- If you're mildly active over the course of your day, you're a 1.2. People who fall into this category include housewives, retail sales people, etc., basically folks who are on their feet throughout the day but not exerting themselves as a part of their jobs (though some moms among you might argue with me on this one).
- If you're active and on your feet, moving at a fast pace, you're a 1.3. I fall into this category, as do most trainers. So might a delivery person, an electrician, a waiter or waitress, basically anyone who's always up, moving around, and exerting energy.
- If you're extremely physically active, you're a 1.4. Construction workers, professional athletes, essentially anyone who is constantly exerting themselves throughout the course of their day would fall into this category.

Once you have identified which category you best fit into, take that number and multiply it by your BMR. So, for example, if my BMR is 1,300 and I consider myself active, I would multiply 1,300 by 1.3 and arrive at 1,690 calories.

3. Calculate your exercise expenditure. Next, you need to address your exercise activity. This one is tough to get perfectly accurate without a heart rate monitor that tracks calories. But if you're training the way I instruct you to in our exercise chapter, then we can guesstimate pretty closely.

- If you're female, you'll burn an additional ten calories for every minute that you train.
- If you're male, you'll burn an additional fifteen calories per minute.

So on the days you exercise, you'll factor in that additional calorie burn from working out. For example, let's say I added thirty minutes of training to my day (which would be thirty minutes x ten calories per minute). That means I burned 300 calories during that time, so I add that to 1,690 and get just about 2,000 calories.

That final number is your AMR, or your active metabolic rate.

4. Decide on your goal. Now that you have your AMR—and a solid idea of how much energy your body is using on a daily basis—it's time to identify your goal to determine how much you should be eating. While this isn't a weight-loss book, we do need to get you to a healthy weight if you're not yet at one, so select which of the following best applies to you.

- You have more than twenty pounds to lose.
- You want to lose vanity weight (i.e., your body is healthy, but you want a different physical aesthetic)—five to fifteen pounds.
- You have no weight to lose and want to look and feel your best.
- You want to gain some weight in a healthy way.

5. Understand the true meaning of calorie restriction. There's just one last thing you need to know, and that's the simple math of calories in and calories out—and what it means for you.

- Calorie deprivation is when you're eating less than your body burns in a day. Simply put, it's Food Intake < Body Burn = Weight Loss.
- Calorie restriction is when you're at a draw with your calorie intake. You aren't eating more or less than what your body burns in a day. Essentially, you're eating as close to your daily AMR burn rate as possible. Simply put, it's Food Intake = Body Burn = Healthy Weight Maintenance.
- Calorie surplus is when you're eating more calories than your body burns in a day. Simply put, it's Food Intake > Body Burn = Weight Gain.

Now, all that said, here's your magic number when it comes to how many calories to eat each day.

If you have more than twenty pounds to lose: You will eat to stay in calorie-deprivation mode.

- Women should eat roughly 1,200 calories a day (with unlimited green vegetables).

- Men should eat roughly 1,600 calories a day (with unlimited green vegetables).

This is a safe calorie floor unless you're morbidly obese and under medical supervision. Then, you may be instructed by your doctor to eat less, but never less than 800 calories a day for women and 1,200 for men (with unlimited green vegetables).

If you have vanity pounds to lose (five to fifteen pounds): You will also eat to remain in calorie-deprivation mode. However, you will only eat 500 calories *less* than your AMR. So, if my AMR is 2,000 calories, then I would eat 1,500 a day. Once you hit your goal weight, you'll begin consuming the same number of calories that you burn daily (your AMR).

This is because wanting to lose vanity pounds and needing to lose visceral fat for health are VERY different beasts. The actual term *vanity pounds* implies that you are perfectly healthy, and your desire to lose weight is purely about aesthetics. Well, your body doesn't share this opinion, and it likes to have a few pounds of fat for perceived purposes of survival. So if you have too large of a calorie deficit and your body is already healthy and at a healthy weight, it will perceive that you are starving and create biochemical shifts to put you in hibernation mode (fat storage, lower energy, etc.). This applies to men and women. (By the way, that is the top reason people plateau with their weight loss.)

Conversely, if you have actual weight to lose for your health, your body handles this very differently. It wants to drop the excess fat and find its equilibrium. That's why different rules apply depending on your goals and needs.

If you have no weight to lose: You will eat to stay in calorie-restriction mode, which means you will eat the exact same number of calories that your body burns over the course of a day.

If you eat less than that and put yourself in calorie deprivation (when you have no stored energy in the form of fat), you're starving your body of proper nutrients. You aren't giving it enough energy, vitamins, minerals, and macros (protein, fat, and carbs) to run properly.

If you have weight you want to gain: You will eat to stay in calorie-surplus mode, but with one important guideline: I don't want you to eat more than your AMR plus 10 percent.

So on a non-exercise day, if my AMR is 1,690, I would only eat an extra 170 calories (bringing my total to 1,860 calories). On an exercise day, when my AMR is 2,000 calories, I would eat 200 extra calories, bringing me to 2,200 calories total. If you eat more than 10 percent, then you increase your risk of building less muscle and storing more fat. Plus, it's simply too much oxidative stress on the body. Once you hit your target weight, you'll begin consuming the same number of calories that you burn daily (your AMR).

WHEN SHOULD YOU EAT?

Over the years, when it comes to the timing of when you should consume your calories, we have gone to both extremes: from eating all day to eating once a day. Again, the answer is in the middle. You're getting sick of hearing that, right? It's pretty simple and straightforward.

- Eat four meals a day: breakfast, lunch, a snack, then dinner.
- Split the three main meals up by three to four hours.
- Divide your AMR among those meals as follows (and don't panic if you aren't spot on; this is optimal, but not essential):
  - Breakfast: 30 percent

- Lunch: 30 percent
- Snack: 10 percent
- Dinner: 30 percent

- Create a minimum of a twelve-hour fast and a maximum of a fifteen-hour fast each day. For example, if you eat every three hours, you will have a fifteen-hour fast between dinner and breakfast. If you eat every four hours, you will have a twelve-hour fast between dinner and breakfast. Personally, I do my best eating every 3.5 hours, with a fourteen-hour fast between dinner and breakfast.

This eating schedule does everything we discussed in the 6 Keys chapters, from managing insulin levels to optimizing your nutrient-sensing pathways to optimizing autophagy (the breaking down of those senescent cells).

In my opinion, there is no need for periods of extreme fasting. They only put you in calorie-deprivation mode, and as I mentioned earlier, if you don't have weight to lose, that means starvation mode. What that mode can cause is what's known in my line of work as refeeding syndrome. What's that? When your body thinks it's starving, it starts breaking down healthy tissue, like muscle, for fuel and throws your entire biochemistry out of whack. Your thyroid hormone levels get messed up and your cortisol goes through the roof, for example, all in an attempt to slow down your BMR. This is what happens on a yo-yo diet.

Finally, you should NOT have binge/cheat days. We've touched upon some of the negative effects of binge days — and even binge meals — in the 6 Keys. They are not healthy, mentally or physically, and are the antithesis of balanced.

WHAT YOU SHOULDN'T EAT

Last, but definitely not least, is the quality of your food. For years now, I've been trying to get people to avoid crap in their food that, in fact, isn't food. My hope is that at this point, that information has reached critical mass. You have hopefully made efforts to adopt this rule of healthy eating. That said, I would be remiss if I didn't give you the recap on what to steer clear of before we jump into what you need to eat. To allow every key to unlock your true potential for healthy aging, you should avoid the following.

Trans fat (aka hydrogenated oil)

Found in: margarine, chips and crackers, baked goods, most fast foods, and certain processed foods made with either margarine or partially hydrogenated vegetable oils.

Trans fat is used to extend the shelf life of food products and is among the most dangerous substances that you can consume. Numerous studies show that trans fats increase LDL (bad) cholesterol levels and decrease HDL (good) cholesterol; increase the risk of heart attacks, heart disease, and strokes; and contribute to inflammation, diabetes, and other health problems.

High fructose corn syrup (aka corn sugar)

Found in: most processed foods, breads, candy, flavored yogurts, salad dressings, canned vegetables, and cereals.

High fructose corn syrup (or HFCS) is a highly refined sweetener that has become the number one source of calories in America. It is found in almost all processed foods. HFCS packs on the pounds faster than any other ingredient, increases your LDL cholesterol levels, and contributes to the development of obesity, diabetes, and tissue damage, among other harmful effects.

Artificial sweeteners (aka sucralose, aspartame, saccharin, etc.)

Found in: most diet or sugar-free foods like soda, desserts, sugar-free gum, drink mixes, baked goods, sweeteners, cereal, breath mints, even chewable vitamins and toothpaste.

These chemicals are known neurotoxins and carcinogens, and account for more reports of adverse reactions than all other foods and food additives combined. In addition to negatively impacting intelligence and short-term memory, artificial sweeteners may also lead to a wide variety of ailments, including brain tumors, lymphoma, diabetes, multiple sclerosis, Parkinson's, Alzheimer's, fibromyalgia, chronic fatigue, emotional disorders like depression and anxiety attacks, dizziness, headaches, nausea, mental confusion, migraines, and seizures.

Artificial colors (red 40, yellow 5 and 6, blue 1 and 2, etc.)

Found in: candy, beverages, cereal, cheese, bakery products, ice cream — basically anything that's either not its original color or seems brighter than it should be.

They're put in there for a reason, and that's to make bad food seem more desirable so you eat more of it. But food coloring has been linked to everything from ADHD to chromosomal damage to thyroid cancer.

Sodium nitrites and nitrates

Found in: hot dogs, bacon, ham, lunch meat, cured meats, corned beef, smoked fish, or any other type of processed meat.

Used as a preservative, coloring, and flavoring, nitrites and nitrates are highly carcinogenic. Once ingested, they form a variety of nitrosamine compounds that enter your bloodstream and wreak havoc on a number of internal organs— your liver and pancreas in particular.

Growth hormones (such as RBST, BGH, etc.)

Found in: non-organic dairy and meat.

These hormones are given to dairy cows and feed-lot cows— either to boost their milk production or to fatten them up for slaughter at an extremely accelerated pace. They may help cows grow, but they also help you age. Studies have linked consumption of these growth hormones to obesity and some forms of cancer, for example.

MSG (aka monosodium glutamate)

Found in: Chinese food, snacks, chips, cookies, seasonings, soup products, frozen dinners, and lunch meats.

This amino acid used as a flavor enhancer is a known excitotoxin—a substance that overexcites cells to the point of damage or death. Studies have shown that it affects the neurological pathways of the brain and may result in adverse side effects, including depression, disorientation, eye damage, fatigue, headaches, and obesity.

Butylated hydroxyanisole (BHA) and butylated hydroxytoluene (BHT)

Found in: potato chips, gum, cereal, frozen sausages, vegetable oils, enriched rice, lard, shortening, candy, and Jell-O.

These two common preservatives keep foods from changing

color, changing flavor, or becoming rancid. But they also affect the neurological system of the brain, alter behavior, and have the potential to cause cancer. That's because both BHA and BHT are oxidants that disrupt the endocrine system and form cancer-causing reactive compounds in your body.

Antibiotics

Found in: livestock.

Antibiotics are given routinely to farm animals to fight infections from inhumane feed-lot conditions and to spur faster-than-normal growth. But they affect not only the animal they're used on but also the human who eats it.

Remember when I discussed how crucial gut health is to overall health and longevity? Well, we know that antibiotics actually kill the good bacteria in our gut—the ones that help us absorb vitamins and minerals. When we can't absorb micronutrients as efficiently, we can't effectively synthesize hormones. This creates an endless list of potential concerns. Beyond just obesity, overuse of antibiotics is causing a massive threat to humanity by creating "superbugs" that are resistant to antibiotics. Overuse is also linked to yeast infections, leaky gut syndrome, candida, and more. You can avoid this by going organic with your meat as often as possible.

Pesticides

Found in: the majority of non-organic fruits and vegetables (particularly thin-skinned varieties and leafy greens).

Pesticides disrupt your endocrine system, which in turn causes your metabolism to malfunction and increases your risk of infertility and cancer, among other things. Fungicides, herbicides, and pesticides are poison. Plain and simple. And the stress these chemicals place on your body and the 6 Keys in particular is tremendous, so avoid them at all costs.

WHAT YOU SHOULD EAT

Now let's address your macronutrient ratio (protein, fat, carbs) and the quality of those macronutrients.

First, you need all three macronutrients for optimal health, and any diet that claims you don't is not only wrong, it's bad for you—it ages you. Period. Remember when we discussed macromolecules? Your cells are made up of all three macronutrients, and when you cut one out, you're literally starving your cells and inviting dysfunction into your body's processes.

Quantity

So we now know how many calories you should be consuming. But how many of those calories should be fat, how many should be protein, and how many should be carbs? In a perfect world your macronutrient ratio for each meal would be as follows:

- **25 to 30 percent fat**
- **30 to 40 percent protein**
- **30 to 40 percent carbohydrates**

Now, if you're thinking the above math doesn't add up, the point is that you can have slightly more carbs than protein one day and have slightly more fat than carbs on another. You don't have to be perfect. It's arguable that there is a perfect ratio anyway, since some people seem to have more energy with a bit more protein and/or fats, and others do better with a little bit more carbs in their diet—and so on. Plus, I have found over the years that when people have to count macros, it makes them a bit nuts. The bottom line: make sure to get a balance of protein, fat, and carbs at every meal.

Quality

The last piece to discuss is the quality of your macronutrients. There are absolutely good and bad categories for each that can either help or hurt your 6 Keys.

Fats: The current trend in nutrition is that fat is your friend, and it absolutely is. But, like all relationships, it's only beneficial with boundaries in place. We've discussed all the incredible benefits that the right fats in the right amount can have on the 6 Keys, from reducing pro-inflammatory cytokines associated with chronic inflammation to lowering cortisol and protecting your telomeres. We've also covered why you must moderate your fat consumption, since too much dietary fat, no matter how healthy it may be for you, can cause an imbalance in gut flora, mess with your epigenome, and promote obesity.

Once again, our theme of balance prevails. Here are the guidelines for healthy fat consumption.

- Avoid consumption of fake fats: trans fats/hydrogenated oils and fractionated oils (such as fractionated coconut oil or fractionated palm oil). If you see any of the above mentioned on the list of ingredients, then skip it.
- Limit consumption of saturated fats such as butter, cream, and other dairy, as well as pork, beef, lamb, and poultry with skin from animals fed corn or soy.
- Limit consumption of palm oil and palm kernel oil.

- Focus on foods rich in polyunsaturated omega-3 fatty acids and monounsaturated fats, such as:
  - **Nuts and seeds:** walnuts, chia, flax, hemp, sunflower, almonds, poppy, hazelnuts, and brazil nuts
  - **Grains:** quinoa and wild rice
  - **Veggies and fruits:** Brussels sprouts, kale, spinach, watercress, avocado, and olives/olive oil
  - **Meat, fish, eggs, and dairy:** wild salmon, mackerel, herring, trout, sardines, anchovies, white fish, grass-fed beef, elk, bison, free-range omega-3 enriched eggs, grass-fed butter, and grass-fed yogurt

Animal protein: Protein has tremendous health benefits, as we discussed throughout the 6 Keys chapters. And it's true that there are plant-based sources of protein that are excellent for you. However, being completely vegan greatly increases your risk of nutrient deficiency, especially of vitamin B12, various forms of collagens, heme iron (which only comes from animals), zinc, calcium, and omega-3 fatty acids.

Again, balance is key. Following are guidelines for consumption of animal protein.

- Go organic with your meat and dairy to avoid hormones and antibiotics.
- Choose meat that is ethically sourced and humane.
- Eat less meat. I recommend absolutely no more than once a day. We don't need nearly as much meat as most Western populations consume. Honestly, I don't eat meat more than four times a week max—and even that is a lot.
- When selecting seafood, avoid chemical additives and absorbed mercury by eating seafood only as often as recommended.

Once a week:

- Halibut, Pacific
- Sablefish (aka black cod), Alaska or Canada
- Tuna, albacore (aka white); canned or fresh; United States or Canada

Twice a Week:

- Catfish, United States
- Caviar, United States, farmed
- Char, Arctic, farmed
- Clams, farmed
- Crab, Dungeness and stone
- Herring, Atlantic
- Mackerel, Atlantic
- Mussels, farmed
- Salmon, wild Alaskan
- Scallops, bay, farmed
- Shrimp, United States, farmed
- Striped bass, farmed
- Sturgeon, farmed
- Tilapia, United States
- Trout, rainbow, farmed

Once a Month:

- Basa or tra (aka catfish), Vietnam
- Clams, wild
- Cod, Pacific

- Crab, blue
- Crab, king, United States
- Crab, snow (aka tanner)
- Flounder and sole, Pacific
- Lobster, American or Maine
- Mahi-mahi
- Sablefish (aka black cod); California, Oregon, or Washington
- Salmon, wild; California, Oregon, or Washington
- Scallops, sea; New England or Canada
- Shrimp, northern, United States
- Shrimp, wild, Canada
- Squid
- Swordfish, United States
- Tilapia, Latin America
- Tuna, albacore (aka white), canned, imported
- Tuna, light, canned
- Tuna, yellowfin (aka ahi), United States

Best to Avoid:

- Caviar, imported, wild
- Chilean sea bass
- Cod, Atlantic
- Crab, king, imported
- Crawfish, China
- Flounder and sole, Atlantic
- Grouper
- Haddock
- Halibut, Atlantic
- Monkfish

- Orange roughy
- Rockfish, Pacific
- Salmon, farmed or Atlantic
- Shark
- Shrimp and prawns, imported
- Skate
- Snapper, red
- Swordfish, imported
- Tilapia, Asia
- Tuna, bluefin
- Tuna, yellowfin (aka ahi), imported

Carbohydrates: Boy, has this macronutrient been raked over the coals in the last twenty years. Mind you, it's absolutely essential to our overall health. The key is to select carbohydrates that don't spike the hell out of your blood sugar and subsequently activate your pancreas to dump insulin into your system.

And while I would love to just give you a chart like the glycemic index to work from, unfortunately, it just isn't that simple. The glycemic index is a tool that tells you how quickly a food breaks down into blood sugar. Theoretically, the faster a food breaks down, the worse it is for you. However, the glycemic index doesn't take into account the amount of carbohydrates or the micronutrients in your food.

For example, according to the glycemic index, a carrot would be considered bad for you because the sugar in it breaks down quickly. But there are two other factors to consider—there is actually very little carbohydrate content in a carrot, and it's loaded with fiber and healthy micronutrients your body needs, such as beta-carotene; vitamins A, B, and C; copper; manganese; calcium; etc.

So, you see there's more to it. But having been in this field a heck of a long time, I'm gonna make this one as simple for you as possible. Below is a list of good carbs and bad carbs to take all the guesswork out of the equation. And remember, if you aren't eating more than your required number of calories and you're working good carbs into each meal with proteins and fats, you'll automatically keep your blood sugar in check and insulin levels stable.

Good Carbs

• Whole grains: great choices include quinoa, millet, oats, whole-grain breads, whole-grain pastas, and whole-grain cereals
• All beans and legumes
• All vegetables: yes, even starches like sweet potatoes, artichokes, and yucca
• All fruits: yes, all of them, as long as you're eating them in their natural form and not canned or dried

Bad Carbs

• All processed grains, such as white flour, enriched flour, white rice, white pasta, pretzels, and cookies
• All processed corn and soy products, such as processed chips and crackers
• All processed sugar, such as white sugar, cakes, cookies, candy, ice cream, and fruit juice

There you have it. Pretty simple, right? All you need to do is eat food in its most natural and unprocessed form, and you're winning.

I'm sure you're wondering if you were meant to go through life without ever eating a croissant or slice of pizza again.

Obviously, these foods aren't ideal, but you can have them per the following guidelines: no more than 20 percent of your daily calories should come from foods that aren't great for you. So if you have 1,800 calories daily, you would have around 360 calories for a slice of pizza, a croissant, etc., but no room for both. And when you eat these foods, opt for organic versions whenever possible. The body can manage sugar in moderation, but things like trans fats and food coloring are always a no.

Alcohol: This is an interesting one because alcohol isn't a protein, fat, or carb—it's literally its own source of fuel. And for years I have said to avoid alcohol. You know all the reasons why: it inhibits fat metabolism, it's loaded with calories, and it's linked to a variety of cancers when overconsumed. However, in moderation, it's also been shown to benefit the 6 Keys. In order to reap the benefits and avoid the dangers, stick to the following ground rules when it comes to alcohol consumption.

- Have no more than two drinks a night.
- Have no more than six drinks a week.
- Avoid sugary, high-calorie beverages (like rum and Cokes and margaritas).
- Steer toward dark alcohol in order to reap the benefits of the antioxidants and polyphenols they contain. Good examples are red wine, dark beer, and whiskey.

Super foods: Yes, there is such a thing as a super food, and we have discussed many of them throughout the 6 Keys chapters. They help create healthier gut flora, lower cortisol, protect our telomeres, etc.

Many believe there must be some special, life-giving

ingredient in these foods. They do give life, but there is no special ingredient. These foods are nutritionally dense and higher in certain essential vitamins and minerals, prebiotic fiber, probiotics, digestive enzymes, omega-3 fatty acids, and polyphenols. We need all of the above for optimal health, beauty, and longevity. The foods, herbs, and spices I list below are simply higher in those nutrients. They are antioxidant-rich foods loaded with omega-3 fatty acids, vitamins, minerals, amino acids, digestive enzymes, probiotics, prebiotics, and polyphenols and should be consumed as often as possible:

Super vegetables rich in polyphenols, minerals, vitamins, and prebiotic fiber

- Leafy greens (organic whenever possible): all, especially spinach, kale, watercress, chard, arugula, and romaine
- Cruciferous vegetables (cooked, not raw): all, particularly Brussels sprouts, broccoli, and cauliflower
- Fungi/mushrooms: reishi, shiitake, oyster, porcini, maitake, chanterelle, white button, and chaga
- Peppers: all, including bell peppers, cayenne peppers, and banana peppers
- Squash: all, including zucchini, butternut, kabocha, spaghetti, and pumpkin
- Root vegetables (organic whenever possible): all, including carrots, beets, parsnips, sweet potatoes, and turnips
- Alliums: all, including garlic, onions, and leeks

Super fruits rich in polyphenols, minerals, vitamins, prebiotic fiber, and enzymes

- Citrus: all, including oranges, limes, lemons, and grapefruit

- Stone fruit (organic whenever possible): all, including cherries, peaches, plums, and apricots
- Berries (organic whenever possible): all, including raspberries, blueberries, kiwi, acai, blackberries, tomatoes, pineapple, and grapes
- Melon: all, including watermelon, cantaloupe, and honeydew
- Other fruits: papaya, pomegranate, pitaya/dragon fruit, mango, apples, pears, quince, and olives

Super nuts and seeds rich in prebiotic fiber and omega-3 fatty acids

- Walnuts
- Almonds
- Hemp
- Flax
- Hazelnuts
- Pecans
- Sunflower
- Chia
- Poppy
- Sesame

Super fermented foods (richer in probiotics)

- Kimchi
- Organic yogurt
- Kefir
- Miso
- Tempeh
- Lassi

Super whole grains rich in prebiotic fiber, vitamins, minerals, and amino acids

- Quinoa
- Millet
- Buckwheat
- Oats
- Bulgur

Super beans and legumes rich in prebiotic fiber, vitamins, and minerals

- Chickpeas
- Kidney beans
- Black beans

Super animal proteins rich in omega-3 fatty acids and amino acids

- Cold-water fish (such as wild salmon, mackerel, and sardines)
- Grass-fed beef, venison, bison, and elk
- Organic free-range omega-3 enriched eggs

Super herbs, spices, and teas rich in vitamins, minerals, and polyphenols

(Cook, supplement, or make tea with the following, but choose organic whenever possible.)

- Ginger
- Rosemary
- Oregano
- Dill

- Ginseng
- Ashwaganda
- Astragalus
- Milk thistle
- Dandelion
- Holy basil
- Cilantro
- Black tea
- Matcha green tea
- Cayenne
- Cloves
- Nutmeg
- Cinnamon
- Turmeric/curcumin
- Black pepper
- Saffron

Miscellaneous

- Red wine: follow the alcohol guidelines established earlier in this chapter and don't overconsume
- Cacao nibs; dark chocolate is also an option, but no more than 100 calories or so daily (two squares) because of the sugar content
- Organic cold-brew coffee: no more than 400 milligrams of caffeine a day (two strong cups)
- Algae: all kinds, especially blue-green algae, spirulina, and chlorella

Supplements: We've got one more topic to discuss, and that's supplements. It's true that in a perfect world, you would get all your nutrients from food, but as I mentioned earlier on, this can be challenging. Our diets might not be varied enough, we might not like certain types of foods, or the soil that our food is grown in may be depleted.

It's definitely easy to get carried away with supplements, but that can be extremely tedious, potentially dangerous, and expensive. If you're so inclined, below are my supplement recommendations for keeping your micronutrient/antioxidant baseline optimal without going overboard. But always get your doctor's permission before taking supplements of any kind.

Omega-3 fish/krill oil: If you don't like fish or don't eat enough of it, consider supplementing with an omega-3 oil. Spend the money on a quality brand in order to avoid any garbage in the product. The true test: Put your supplement in the refrigerator. If it becomes cloudy, it's not high quality.

Brands I like: Alaya Naturals, Barlean's, Ultra Omega-3

Probiotics: If you don't eat fermented foods at least once a week, or if you have recently taken antibiotics, consider taking a probiotic supplement to rebuild and maintain a healthy balance of good gut flora.

Brands I like: Alaya Naturals, Bio-K, Healthy Trinity, Dr. Axe

Grass-fed whey protein powder with branched-chain amino acids (BCAAs): I use this as part of my nutrition plan. I put it in smoothies, cereal, oatmeal, whatever I can. Since I find it hard to get all my aminos in, I love a protein powder with aminos. And if you're vegan or vegetarian, there are some plant-based alternatives with BCAAs. Just look for hemp or pumpkin seed and avoid soy.

Brands I like: Alaya Naturals, Naked Whey, NOW

An organic multivitamin: Multivitamins are a great way to make sure you're getting all your basic vitamins and minerals.

Brands I like: Alaya Naturals, Rainbow, New Chapter, Paradise

A collagen blend: I strongly recommend a collagen supplement unless you drink bone-broth-based soups regularly. It's important to look for a product with all types of collagen in it.

Brands I like: Alaya Naturals, Dr. Axe

A super-antioxidant blend: I also strongly recommend this. I find it dizzying to constantly read about things like chia, maqui berry, noni berry, etc. Personally, I take a super-antioxidant blend to cover my bases.

Brands I like: Alaya Naturals, HealthForce, Sunfood

Greens powder: If you don't eat your greens or eat enough of them, I suggest investing in greens powder. You can also just mix this in with your smoothie or protein shake.

Brands I like: Alaya Naturals, Garden of Life

An adaptogenic herb blend: This is another supplement I take. Mine has ashwaganda, astragalus, turmeric, and cordyceps, to name a few. I take it because I simply don't know how to get most of these ingredients into my food.

Brands I like: Alaya Naturals, Dr. Axe

If you are so inclined you can visit the Alaya Naturals website to learn more about most of these supplements: alayanaturals.com.

So here's our summary of action steps:

- Figure out your active metabolic rate (AMR) and how many calories to eat each day by:
  - Calculating your BMR
  - Figuring out your daily activity score
  - Calculating your exercise expenditure
  - Deciding your goal, whether:
    - You have more than twenty pounds to lose
    - You want to lose vanity weight (five to fifteen pounds)
    - You have no weight to lose and want to look and feel your best
    - You want to gain some weight in a healthy way

- Eat four meals a day: breakfast, lunch, a snack, then dinner
  - Split the main meals up by three to four hours
  - Divide your AMR among those meals as follows
    - Breakfast: 30 percent
    - Lunch: 30 percent
    - Snack: 10 percent
    - Dinner: 30 percent
- Each meal, your macronutrient ratio should break down as follows:
  - 25 to 30 percent fat
  - 30 to 40 percent protein
  - 30 to 40 percent carbohydrates
- Create a minimum of a twelve-hour fast and a maximum of a fifteen-hour fast each day.
- Do not have binge/cheat days.

- Avoid the following:
  - Trans fat, hydrogenated oils, and fractionated oils
  - High fructose corn syrup
  - Artificial sweeteners
  - Artificial colors
  - Sodium nitrites and nitrates
  - Growth hormones
  - MSG
  - Butylated hydroxyanisole (BHA) and butylated hydroxy-toluene (BHT)
  - Antibiotics
  - Pesticides
- Limit consumption of:
  - Saturated fats
  - Palm oil and palm kernel oil
  - Meat (no more than once a day)

- Focus on foods such as:
  - Walnuts, chia, flax, hemp, sunflower, almonds, poppy-seeds, hazelnuts, and brazil nuts
  - Quinoa and wild rice
  - Brussels sprouts, kale, spinach, watercress, avocado, and olives/olive oil
  - Organic and ethically sourced foods such as wild salmon, mackerel, herring, trout, sardines, anchovies, white fish, grass-fed beef, elk, bison, free-range omega-3 enriched eggs, grass-fed butter, and grass-fed yogurt

- Choose good carbs such as:
  - Whole grains: quinoa, millet, oats, whole-grain breads, whole-grain pastas, and whole-grain cereals

- ○ All beans and legumes
- ○ All fruits and vegetables

- Avoid bad carbs such as:
  - ○ All processed grains
  - ○ All processed corn and soy products
  - ○ All processed sugar

- When drinking alcohol:
  - ○ Have no more than two drinks a night.
  - ○ Have no more than six drinks a week.
  - ○ Avoid sugary, high-calorie beverages.
  - ○ Choose dark alcohols over lighter versions when possible

- When considering supplements, ask your doctor about trying:
  - ○ Omega-3 fish/krill oil
  - ○ Probiotics
  - ○ Grass-fed whey protein powder with branched-chain amino acids
  - ○ An organic multivitamin
  - ○ A collagen blend
  - ○ A super-antioxidant blend
  - ○ Greens powder
  - ○ An adaptogenic herb blend

CHAPTER 14

The 6 Keys Exercise Strategy

People are always looking for a way to get fit without fitness.

Repeat what I just said out loud: fit...without fitness? Seriously?

Sure, some "experts" will try to tell you that with their diet or wellness program, you don't have to work out. It's what they think most people want to hear. But it's BS. I know that to be fact, just as I know that if you've ever tried one of these types of wellness or diet programs, you know it, too. And even if you lose weight by starving it off, you will just put it all back on and then some once you start eating normally again. And, this isn't a weight loss book. It's about aging amazingly and we can't do that without exercise, period.

Getting fit—burning fat, building muscle, and improving your strength and endurance—when done properly, is a veritable fountain of youth. If you want to live long and live well, it's nonnegotiable.

In the past, while I have been labeled things like hard-core and toughest trainer, in truth, I think I have been very forgiving. Do I ask a lot? Yes. But I also try to see where someone is presently, then help them to simply get out and move.

But in this book, I'm asking for a little more. You don't get to

100-plus with your wits about you and your health intact by doing the bare minimum. You just don't. According to the science, turning those 6 Keys with ease means incorporating the right exercise regimen. That will involve the following:

- Working out four to five times a week for at least twenty to thirty minutes
- Lifting weights and/or engaging in bodyweight resistance training
- Training at 80 to 85 percent of your maximum heart rate (MHR)
- Making sure to take one day off per week (preferably two)

I'm going to put all this together for you, but if you want me to literally train you in all these techniques you can check out the 6 Keys exercise program I built into the Jillian Michaels My Fitness App here: https://www.jillianmichaels.com/6keys2app.

THE EXERCISE AND ANTI-AGING EQUATION

Throughout this book, I have referenced specific fitness techniques that positively impact the 6 Keys, such as resistance training, circuit training, and HIIT training. I have promoted these techniques for years. They not only help you age well, but also are very effective at burning fat and building lean muscle.

In a perfect world, I would have you work all three of these forms of fitness training into your week. But first, let's make sure you understand each before we play mix-and-match.

Resistance training: In a nutshell, resistance training is any form of exercise where your muscles are working against something that resists your movement and causes your skeletal muscles to contract. It doesn't matter to your muscles what that something is—they could be resisting against gravity, iron, cables, you name it. It also doesn't matter what kinds of exercises you do—bodyweight exercises (push-ups, pull-ups, etc.), free weights (barbells, dumbbells, or kettlebells, for example), or machine exercises (like a lat pull-down station, a leg-press machine, etc.). It all counts, so long as you're making your muscles work hard enough. The only thing that matters is that you incorporate this type of training into your workouts.

Circuit training: A circuit-training routine is one where you run through a series of strength-training exercises one after the other with little to no rest in between. Ideally, the exercises you choose target every major, and minor, muscle group, so that after you're through, you've worked your entire body from head to toe. But the benefits go beyond a full-body effort. When done right, a good circuit-training routine can improve both muscular strength and endurance.

HIIT: Short for high-intensity interval training, this exercise technique alternates periods of short, intense all-out activity with less intense rest periods. HIIT is one of the most effective fitness techniques when it comes to the 6 Keys, and compared to continuous, steady-state training, there really is no contest— HIIT is the game-changer.

In a pure HIIT workout, you would pick an aerobic activity that works your heart and burns calories—for example, running, biking, stair-climbing, jumping jacks, or skipping rope—and then do it in a very specific way, alternating from a high to a low intensity over and over again, in order to raise your heart rate and the overall intensity.

The intensity-to-recovery ratio time for HIIT can vary. A typical HIIT protocol like Tabata has a 2-to-1 ratio, which means you would exercise as hard as you could for twenty seconds, take a ten-second rest, then repeat this pattern for eight intervals. (Yes, the whole routine lasts only four minutes.) However, this isn't ideal for the average person, and four minutes won't cut it for our purposes. Researchers believe a longer stretch of time is more effective — exercising anywhere from twenty to thirty minutes with any of the following interval ratios: for a beginner, thirty seconds to two minutes with a recovery ratio of 1 to 1 (for example, thirty seconds high/thirty seconds rest); for an intermediate level, 2 to 1 (such as thirty seconds high/fifteen seconds rest); and for an advanced level, 3 to 1 (for example, thirty seconds high/ten seconds rest).

THE AGE-REVERSING FORMULA

Metabolic circuit training (MCT) combines circuit training and resistance training. MCT requires you to perform resistance-training exercises (whether bodyweight moves, free-weight moves, or machines) in swift succession with very little (preferably zero) rest between exercises.

This type of routine isn't perfect just for combating aging; it is ideal from an overall fitness standpoint as well. It stimulates a significantly higher total calorie burn and EPOC (short for excess post-exercise oxygen consumption) compared to continuous, steady-state training and HIIT cardio-only workouts.

How does it do that? There is a direct relationship between exercise intensity and EPOC, which is the amount of oxygen it takes to bring your body back to a normal metabolic state after intense exercise. Sure, you may feel fine minutes after an intense workout, but your body has to rebuild damaged tissues, rebalance the oxygen levels in your blood, restore stored glycogen, and handle a few other tasks. All that work takes energy and oxygen, causing you to burn significantly more calories for twenty-four to forty-eight hours afterward. The more you raise the intensity, the harder your body has to work to consume more oxygen and restore itself.

In fact, MCT produces a greater EPOC response than traditional resistance-training routines and burns approximately twice the number of calories. You'll also be doing HIIT intervals in between MCT circuits, because doing both further enhances EPOC, as long as the intensity is high enough. This combination allows you to turn all 6 Keys in the right direction.

Ideally, I would suggest doing four MCT sessions a week for a minimum of twenty minutes to a maximum of forty minutes (as well as a five-minute warm-up and five-minute cool-down). In addition, you'll perform either one HIIT workout or two low-intensity cardio workouts in between. For example, your weekly workout regimen might look like this:

- On Mondays and Thursdays, your MCT workouts focus on your PUSH muscles (chest, shoulders, triceps, quadriceps, and core).
- On Tuesdays and Fridays, your MCT workouts focus on your PULL muscles (back, biceps, hamstrings, glutes, and core).
- On Wednesdays and Saturdays, you do either a longer duration, lower-intensity cardio workout on both days, or a pure HIIT workout on one of the two days (but only one day, not both).
- Sunday is (and must be) a complete day of rest.

Here is just one idea of how you could incorporate MCT circuits using nothing but bodyweight exercises:

Mondays and Thursdays (PUSH muscles)

Push-ups
Squats
Dips
Forward lunges
HIIT—burpees
[Do each move for thirty seconds before moving to the next.
Rest one minute between circuits. Repeat for two rounds.]

Tuesdays and Fridays (PULL muscles)

Pull-ups or assisted pull-ups
Step-ups
Body rows
Alternating side lunges
HIIT—butt kicks
[Do each move for thirty seconds before moving to the next.
Rest one minute between circuits. Repeat for two rounds.]

Here's another MCT circuit that uses nothing but free-weight exercises:

Mondays and Thursdays (PUSH muscles)

Squat thrusts (with barbell)
Weighted dead lifts
Chest flies with leg raises
Sumo squats with triceps extensions
HIIT—jumping jacks

[Do each move for thirty seconds before moving to the next.
Rest one minute between circuits. Repeat for two rounds.]

Tuesdays and Fridays (PULL muscles)

Lat pull-downs
Stiff leg / Romanian dead lifts
Dumbbell rows
Weighted pelvic thrusts
HIIT—jumping rope
[Do each move for thirty seconds before moving to the next.
Rest one minute between circuits. Repeat for two rounds.]

On Wednesdays and Saturdays, you'll hit cardio by doing a lower-intensity activity (such as light hiking, a spin class, swimming, etc.) for forty-five to sixty minutes. But ideally, one of your cardio days should be a HIIT day; your goal should be a twenty-five-minute workout (including a five-minute cardio warm-up).

First, pick an aerobic exercise: running, biking, swimming, jumping rope, rowing, stair-climbing, etc. You can even experiment with bodyweight exercises such as squat jumps, jumping jacks, speed skating, mountain climbing, butt kicks, or high knees, for example.

Second, decide what level you consider yourself to be, then follow these recommendations:

• If you're a **beginner,** train with a 1-to-1 ratio. Exercise at a high intensity for thirty seconds, recover for thirty seconds by exercising at a low intensity (50 percent of your maximum effort), then repeat this sequence over twenty-five minutes.

- If you're **intermediate,** train with a 2-to-1 ratio. Exercise at a high intensity for thirty seconds, recover for fifteen seconds by exercising at a low intensity, then repeat this sequence over twenty-five minutes.
- Finally, if you're **advanced,** train with a 3-to-1 ratio. Exercise at a high intensity for thirty seconds, recover for just ten seconds by exercising at a low intensity, then repeat this sequence over twenty-five minutes — this one is brutal.

BTW: The duration of time to plug into those ratios can vary. Like everything else, variety is key. I would say that most of the time, you should keep your intervals at anywhere from twenty seconds minimum to one minute maximum. But if you wanted to push yourself once a month or so with two-minute intervals, you absolutely could.

How much is too much?

In terms of resistance training, the big question people often have is how much weight they should lift and how many times they should lift it. There really isn't a wrong answer, but there are guidelines.

First, the amount of resistance should have an inverse relationship to the number of repetitions you do. The more weight that you're lifting, the fewer repetitions you'll be able to do. Conversely, the less weight you're lifting, the more repetitions you'll be able to do. Both ways to train are equally important because they achieve different goals. More weight/fewer reps helps build muscular strength, while less weight/more reps builds muscular endurance. Changing things up helps you gain all the benefits of resistance training.

THE FOUR TENETS

There are **four tenets** that must be adhered to if you hope to reap all the potential benefits that fitness holds for the 6 Keys: intensity, progression/variety, recovery, and consistency.

When you apply these tenets, you can create the most effective, efficient, powerful training regimen possible. They also keep your workouts from becoming boring. You may not love what I have to say, but if you follow these tenets, your life will change dramatically.

1. Intensity

Proper intensity is arguably the most important pillar of your training. Ideally it's gauged by your maximum heart rate (MHR)—the upper threshold of what your cardiovascular system can handle during physical activity. If you don't push yourself hard enough, you won't see longevity-extending results.

What's your ideal heart rate? Well, it depends on the workout. Intensity has an inverse relationship to exercise duration. So the less time you have to sweat, the harder your training should be, and vice versa.

For example, you could hike for several hours at 60 to 65 percent of your MHR. Or you could do a thirty-minute exercise session with me that consisted of resistance training and HIIT intervals, and your heart rate would jump to about 85 percent of your MHR.

What's the better option? When it comes to combating age, the more effective workout is a shorter-duration, higher-intensity HIIT session.

The reason I'm asking you to do longer cardio workouts at a

lower intensity is that I'm sure you'll still want to do them because they're fun. I do things like hike with my dogs and paddleboard or snowboard with my kids. And while these types of lower-intensity activities aren't the *most* effective at age-proofing your life, they are still far better than nothing.

On your MCT days, you want to be working out at an intensity of around 80 to 85 percent of your maximum heart rate. To figure that number—and how to attain it—simply **subtract your age from the number 220.**

For example, since I'm 44 years old, my MHR is 220 − 44 = 176 beats per minute. So when I do MCT, I try to keep my heart rate at around 80 to 85 percent of that number. Eighty percent would be .80 x 176, or 141 beats a minute; 85 percent would be .85 x 176, or 150 beats a minute. So I shoot to keep my heart rate at around 145 beats a minute.

A heart rate monitor is helpful, but you don't need one to track this. All you have to do is stop and count your heartbeats for six seconds during training and then multiply by ten. I know that I need my heart to beat fourteen to fifteen times every six seconds in order to be at 140 to 150 beats a minute.

So a beginner who is the same age as a world-class athlete might have the same target heart rate. Why? Advanced athletes are better conditioned, so they need to work out at a far greater intensity to reach the same heart rate as a beginner.

For example, if you're the same age as Serena Williams (and not a world-class athlete), you might only need to run eight-mile-per-hour sprints with no incline to reach the same heart rate as Serena does when she runs sprints at twelve miles per hour with a 10 percent incline.

Why do I bring this up? Because as you become fitter, you'll need to adjust the intensity of your workouts in order to hit your target heart rate.

2. Progression and Variety

Remember that exercise is stress, and your body responds to that stress by adapting to it and becoming fitter, stronger, and healthier. However, if you do the same things at the gym all the time, then two things happen. One, your body adapts to the point where it stops progressing. Two, you run the risk of injury by overusing certain muscles, joints, and so forth, especially if you don't incorporate the appropriate recovery strategies (another principle I'll get to in a moment).

Progression and variety, while different from each other, work hand in hand to deliver certain intersecting benefits.

Progression

Aim to intensify your workouts every two weeks by roughly 10 percent. What does that mean? You could:

- Add 10 percent more weight to an exercise.
- Do 10 percent more repetitions.
- Rest 10 percent less between exercises or between sets.

Overall, the goal is for you to constantly challenge yourself with slightly more advanced fitness targets. As long as you always maintain a heart rate that's 80 to 85 percent of your MHR, you'll be pushing yourself with the right amount of intensity as your body becomes stronger.

Variety

Variety in your workouts is just as crucial as progression. You need to work your body in different ways in order to maximize your strength, agility, balance, and flexibility.

You could simply perform a more difficult version of an exercise you're presently doing, for instance, taking a regular squat and making it a jump squat. Or you could vary what I call the FOCs, or factors of change.

Before you try to change, though, it's imperative you master the basics so that you create a strong foundation.

Range of motion: By moving through a full range of motion in your exercises, you will gain more flexibility, mobility, and strength, and burn more calories. Your range of motion might be limited if you do, for example:

- A squat where you fail to bring your thighs parallel to the ground
- A biceps curl or lat pull-down where you never fully release the weight back to the start position or straighten your arms
- A lunge where the rear knee comes to about six inches from the floor instead of two inches
- A military dumbbell press where you never fully straighten your arms overhead

As you perform any exercise, ask yourself: am I going as far up or down as I safely could be? Of course, if you're extremely tight and can't get all the way there, don't injure yourself trying. But if you are mindlessly moving through your workout, phoning it in, or just not pushing hard enough, stop cheating yourself. Moving your body those few extra inches will increase your fitness quickly and effectively.

Levers: Your limbs are levers, and the farther away they are from the center of your body, your core, the harder your muscles have to work to raise or lower a weight.

Here's the best-known example: beginners are often told to do push-ups on their hands and knees instead of their hands and feet. This is because flopping to your knees shortens the levers of your legs, thereby decreasing the resistance and making the exercise easier.

Your goal should be to use levers to help you progress in your workout and gradually increase your intensity. So if you're doing a lateral shoulder raise with your arms bent, work up to having them extended to increase the lever length. If you're doing push-ups on your knees, work up to push-ups on your hands and feet.

Speed: The best way to make an adjustment to your workout is to change the tempo or speed. For our purposes, speed is applied in two ways:

1. HIIT intervals: no matter which aerobic exercise you choose for your HIIT workouts, you can increase the intensity simply by increasing how fast you perform the exercise.
2. Resistance training exercises in your MCT program: as you perform each exercise, you can also gradually increase how fast you perform the movement. However, speed should only be applied to what's called the concentric portion of an exercise. This is the part of the movement where the muscle shortens as it

contracts, or in simpler terms, it's the portion where you're raising, pulling, or pushing the weight. It's the pulling part of a
pull-up, the curling part of a biceps curl, and the pushing part of
a push-up. One key caveat: don't use speed for any abs or core
move.

Balance/stability: Ever look around the gym at all the interesting
equipment like pillow discs, Bosu balls, wobble boards, and so on
and wonder how to use them? For our purposes, you really don't
need them. They might be great for rehab but not for anti-aging,
because exercises using these types of balance tools only tend to
decrease your overall power (speed and strength combined) and
build less muscle. And when it comes to staying ageless, you need
all the lean muscle you can get—and keep!

That said, balance training (minus all the fancy balance tools)
does have benefits when done in a way that doesn't compromise
resistance, speed, and power. The key is to stick to exercises performed on a solid surface (aka the floor), then finding ways to
make yourself less stable (but still safe). What do I mean? Instead
of balancing on both feet and/or using both arms during an exercise, try raising an arm or leg up (or off the floor) to create instability. For example:

• Do push-ups with one leg off the ground.
• Do single-leg squats by keeping one foot an inch or so off
the floor.
• Do a single-arm plank by extending one arm out to your
side or in front of you.

The possibilities are endless. Simply assess the exercise you're performing and see if you can safely remove one pillar of support.

Statics: A static is when you stop at some point during an exercise — usually the midpoint of the move — either to perform an isometric contraction (aka flexing your muscles) or to simply pause to keep tension in your muscles.

Using statics during not just basic exercises but also combination exercises (where you perform two exercises at once) can be very effective. For example, you could hold the midpoint position of a lunge while performing shoulder presses, hold the midpoint of a squat while performing biceps curls, or hold the midpoint of a sumo squat while performing triceps extensions. Again, the possibilities are endless.

Plyo: Short for plyometrics, put simply, plyo is jump training — meaning, any exercise that forces you to defy gravity by hopping, bounding, jumping, springing, soaring, and skyrocketing your body off the floor. Plyo training is an extreme form of high-intensity training that can significantly increase your strength, speed, and endurance, allowing you to burn more calories and lose fat.

Here's how it works. You perform a high-velocity movement (like a squat jump) that relies on power generated from what is called the stretch-shortening cycle. A muscle that is stretched before an explosive contraction (called recoil) will contract more forcefully and rapidly. Using a squat jump as our example, squatting down just prior to the jump lowers your center of gravity and slightly stretches the muscles involved. Then as you straighten your legs to jump, you ignite more potential for explosion.

Here are some other examples of plyo movements:

- A lunge in which you jump as you straighten your legs
- A box jump, where you bend your knees, and then jump onto a box or platform
- A push-up where you thrust your upper body vertically from the lowered position with such force that your hands leave the ground

One warning: while the physical benefits of plyo are unsurpassed, this type of training is extremely intense. Do not attempt it unless you are already at a moderate level of fitness. If you have an injury or health condition, be sure to consult with your doctor before engaging in this activity.

3. Recovery

The 6 Keys can work either for you or against you, and exercise is a huge factor in which way that pendulum swings. We know that fitness benefits us when done properly, but what about when it's done wrong? At best, it's minimally helpful at turning all the keys. At worst, it can lead to overtraining, which can cause chronic inflammation, chronic stress, and injury.

There's one way to avoid the pitfalls of too much fitness: it's imperative that you allow enough recovery time. The best game plan:

- Make sure to take at least one day off each week from exercise — preferably two.
- Never train a muscle group *intensely* more than twice a week.
- Make sure to allow forty-eight to seventy-two hours of rest between exercise sessions, particularly the more intense sessions where you're doing heavy resistance training.

How do you do all that and still get at least four thirty-minute workouts in? As I instructed you earlier, by training your push muscles on one day and your pull muscles on another—a technique that uses muscle splits to your advantage.

The reason I prefer to pair muscle groups with primarily the same function together is twofold: it improves recovery by giving your muscles enough time to rest, and it maximizes intensity by thoroughly fatiguing your muscles.

Muscles with the same function (either pulling or pushing) generally work together to perform an exercise. For example, whenever you push something away from you, whether a dumbbell, barbell, kettlebell, or even yourself from the floor, your chest, shoulders, triceps, and/or quadriceps muscles are used to some degree. Whenever you pull something toward you, your back, biceps, and/or hamstring and glute muscles generally work together.

If you don't train muscles with the same function on the same days, it makes it nearly impossible to maximize your strength during your workouts or have enough recovery time afterward. For example, if you did biceps curls on a Monday, but then seated rows for your back muscles (which recruits your biceps, too) on Tuesday, you'd be working your biceps two days in a row, which doesn't give them enough recovery time. In addition, your back workout would suffer because the biceps would be too fatigued from the workout the day before. The schedule I've suggested in this chapter optimizes calorie burn, muscle conditioning, and fat metabolism throughout the week, all the while giving your muscles an opportunity to rest, repair, and rebuild.

Similarly, if you're into exercise classes, think about what muscles they train. For example, if you do yoga on Monday, which by its nature is very chest, shoulders, and triceps intensive (lots of planks, chaturangas, and downward-facing dogs), don't take a boot-camp class full of push-ups, presses, and dips on Tuesday, because you'll be targeting the same muscle groups. Instead, take a class that focuses more on your lower body.

While this might take slightly more planning on your part, I assure you that it's worth the effort and will make an enormous difference in your results.

Finally, the golden rule: never train a muscle if it's still sore from a previous workout.

4. Consistency

Consistency may be the most important tenet. After all, if you follow all of the recommendations I've just thrown out there every single time you sweat, but if you don't train on a regular basis, it doesn't matter. You'll never reap the benefits, and you'll constantly run the risk of injury as your body never properly adapts, progresses, and transforms.

So—stick with it. And if you don't want to give up your favorite boxing gym or yoga class, then incorporate them—just do it strategically. Make your boxing workout your HIIT day, or your yoga workout your push day. You get the gist.

Ultimately, no matter what workout you choose—a boot-camp class, a yoga class, a kickboxing class, or weight training at the gym—get your heart rate up to 80 to 85 percent of your max to ensure maximum key-turning power.

So here's our summary of action steps:

- Incorporate an exercise regimen that involves the following:
  - Working out four to five times a week for at least twenty to thirty minutes

- ○ Lifting weights and/or engaging in bodyweight resistance training
- ○ Training at 80 to 85 percent of your maximum heart rate (MHR)
- Ideally, do four MCT sessions a week for a minimum of twenty minutes to a maximum of forty minutes (including warm-up and cool-down).
- Ideally, perform either one HIIT workout or two low-intensity cardio workouts a week.
- Remember and adhere to the four tenets:
  - ○ **Intensity**—always adjust the intensity of your workouts in order to hit your target heart rate.
  - ○ **Progression/variety**—continuously try new exercises/moves to challenge your body in different ways, and aim to intensify your workouts every two weeks by roughly 10 percent by:
    - Adding 10 percent more weight to an exercise
    - Doing 10 percent more repetitions within a certain amount of time
    - Resting 10 percent less between exercises or between sets
  - ○ **Recovery**—make sure to take at least one day off each week from exercise—preferably two. Also:
    - Never train a muscle group *intensely* more than twice a week.
    - Make sure to allow forty-eight to seventy-two hours of rest between exercise sessions, particularly the more intense sessions.
  - ○ **Consistency**—train on a regular basis and don't let excuses get in the way of your exercise.

CHAPTER 15

The 6 Keys Environment Strategy

In the 6 Keys chapters, we covered some of the damage that environmental toxins do to our health and longevity. In this chapter, I'm going to cover what the heck you can do about it, and how you can mitigate the onslaught of toxins and pollutants that bombard you from all areas in your life.

The journal *Environmental Health Perspectives* reports that well over eighty thousand synthetic chemicals were introduced in the United States from 1952 to 2002, with an additional two to three thousand new chemicals introduced every year since. These chemicals are being dispersed in huge amounts in our air and water, and among our farms, homes, and towns. Scary, right?

To age well and keep your 6 Keys turning smoothly, it's imperative that you do your best to clean up and purify not just the food you eat, but the air you breathe, the water you drink, the products you use to clean your home and your body, the materials you cook with and package your food in, and even the furnishings in your home.

Unfortunately, it isn't possible to remove all of these chemicals, as not all are in our control. But you can eliminate some of them and minimize the rest. Let's start with the air we breathe.

CLEAN UP YOUR INDOOR AIR

According to a study by the California Environmental Protection Agency (EPA), every man, woman, and child exchanges between ten thousand and seventy thousand liters of air every twenty-four hours. So you can see why it's important to keep air as pollutant-free as possible.

When it comes to outdoor air, it's not so easy to change the air you breathe. Sure, you could move to a region with better air quality and stronger regulations on pollutants, but if you don't feel like uprooting, focus on the quality of your indoor air.

Surprisingly, indoor air is far more polluted than outdoor air. According to the EPA, indoor air has on average two to five times as many contaminants as outdoor air—and that number can range as high as 100 times more contaminants. This is true even if you live in a big city. So what makes up all that nasty air?

Airborne bacteria and viruses: These can come from people and pets, damp indoor spaces, and humidifiers and air conditioners that aren't kept clean.

Your best option: Make sure to clean your air ducts and regularly replace air filters, and don't let water sit in humidifiers. And wash your hands often (for at least twenty seconds) to scrub off any airborne contagions that may have landed on things you have touched during the day.

Asbestos: Older buildings can have insulation and soundproofing materials containing asbestos.

Your best option: If you live or work in an environment with asbestos, hire a professional to remove it when you're out of your home or workplace.

Carbon monoxide: This dangerous gas has no color, odor, or taste. Exposure to it can cause headaches, nausea, dizziness, damage to the brain, heart, and central nervous system—and even death. Minute amounts of carbon monoxide are naturally found in our bodies and in the air. Large amounts, however, can be released from cars, furnaces, or other fuel-burning appliances. You can also be exposed from cigarette smoke (first- and second-hand), a fire, or by coming into contact with methylene chloride, found in paint removers and other solvents.

Your best option: Many states require carbon monoxide monitors in private residences, and some also require them in public places. Whether or not they are required in your state, I strongly recommend having one of these, along with a smoke detector, to catch any car exhaust or furnace leaks that might be poisoning your indoor air. The cost is low and the potential to avoid tragedy is high, so get on it.

Product off-gassing: Believe it or not, this is likely the primary cause of indoor air pollution in your home. Have you ever walked into a freshly painted home and been darn near knocked out by the smell? That's because volatile organic compounds, or VOCs, (benzene, ammonia, formaldehyde, kerosene, and a host of other known carcinogens and toxins) are off-gassing.

New carpets, pressed-wood products like particle board and plywood, mattresses, fabrics, glues and adhesives in furniture, and fumes from paint, household cleaners, dry-cleaned clothes, air fresheners, and even home printers and copy machines can all cause major indoor air pollution in the form of VOCs.

According to the EPA, VOCs not only cause irritation to your eyes and respiratory tract but also cause loss of coordination, nausea, and headaches, and can damage vital organs like your liver and kidneys as well as your central nervous system. They have also been shown to cause cancer in animals. Levels of VOCs are typically ten times higher inside than outside. You don't want to mess around with them.

Your best option: Be sure to buy green. How do you do that? Buy natural-fiber throw rugs you can toss into the washing machine. If you decide you must have carpeting, I suggest natural-fiber, eco-friendly materials such as abaca, raffia, or seagrass.

When it comes to furniture, choose solid wood instead of particle board or plywood, and look for items made with natural materials such as bamboo, organic cotton, and naturally tanned leather. And even if it's all-natural, make sure that it's either untreated or treated with natural substances. Synthetic materials or natural materials treated with synthetic substances release chemicals into the air, including VOCs. Instead, look for furniture that is free of:

- PVC
- Formaldehyde-based glues
- Toxic flame retardants
- Wood stains that contain the industrial chemical perfluorooctanoic acid (PFOA)

The next time you paint, make sure to get VOC free, no VOC, or zero VOC paint, which is almost completely free of carcinogenic chemicals. Check out www.afmsafecoat.com. This is the stuff we used in our home. Finally, check out www.greenguard.org. This certifying organization ensures that furniture has a low toxicity; it lists many different suppliers on the website.

Mold: Mold can grow anywhere there's moisture—especially in places where you've had any type of water damage. It can cause allergic reactions, asthma, sinus infections, rashes, upper respiratory infections, and even anemia. The more common types of mold aren't deadly, but one rare type of mold, mycotoxin (known as toxic mold), can cause many serious health complications, including convulsions and even death.

Your best option: If you see or suspect mold, call a professional to test for it. If they find it, have it removed ASAP—this is a job for professionals.

Radon: This cancer-causing, radioactive gas is, like carbon monoxide, undetectable. You can't see, taste, or smell it, yet it's the second highest cause of lung cancer after cigarette smoking! Created naturally from the decay and breakdown of underground uranium, radon can be found in soil, well water, and building materials like granite and cement. It creeps into your house through cracks in your home's foundation or other openings, then gets trapped in there.

Your best option: For peace of mind, get a radon test. You can pay about three hundred dollars to get this done, or you can buy a test kit from a local hardware store for about twenty to thirty dollars and do it yourself. You can also purchase a test online at www.radon.com, www.radon.info, or www.radonmonitor.com.

If you find that your home has high concentrations of radon, don't worry. You can fix most radon problems yourself for less than five hundred dollars—well worth the money. If you require the assistance of a professional, I recommend checking out the list of certified radon mitigators in your state at http://www.radon.com/radon/radon_map.html.

Smoke: Whether from cigarettes or chimneys, automobile exhaust, or even improperly vented heaters, smoke (and the toxic by-products it contains) can be a major indoor air pollutant.

Your best option: Don't smoke, don't be around people who smoke, and seriously reconsider that cozy winter fire. If you must light one, follow the guidelines below:

• Use only untreated wood that has dried out for at least five to six months—it will give off less smoke.

• Use Java-Log fire logs, which are widely available and the least toxic manufactured fire log.

• Have your chimney cleaned and serviced yearly, so there is no buildup of creosote (a wood-tar combination that can cause chimney fires) and toxic smoke doesn't end up filling your living room.

• If you must have a fire, consider switching from a wood-burning fireplace to one that burns natural gas or to a pellet stove.

Lead: I'm sure I don't need to tell you how toxic this stuff is. The EPA has stated that more than 80 percent of the homes built before 1978 likely contain some lead, because it was not banned from paint until that year.

Your best option: If you suspect there might be lead in your home, the National Lead Information Center offers a list of EPA-certified labs near you where you can send paint chips to be tested. They'll also provide you with a list of lead abatement specialists who can seal or remove the lead. Or you can contact www.leadlisting.com. Do *not* try to remove the lead paint yourself! And be sure you and your family are out of the home while it is being removed.

In addition to avoiding or minimizing exposure to these pollutants, there are other things you can do to help improve your indoor air quality:

• Open the windows whenever possible to air out any toxic fumes.

• Get house plants. NASA scientists found that one potted plant for every hundred square feet can help remove harmful contaminants from the air in your home. Best varieties to buy: bamboo, English ivy, gerbera daisy, and green spider.

• Avoid dry-cleaning your clothes. Instead, try a wet cleaner. These guys use cleaner, greener soaps to get the job done. Or try a green dry cleaner. These eco-friendly companies use pressurized carbon dioxide rather than traditional dry-cleaning chemicals. Worst-case scenario, if you must dry-clean your clothes, take them out of the plastic and leave them outside to off-gas for four hours minimum.

• Avoid air fresheners and instead opt for natural soy candles, which aren't toxic.

• Don't store harsh chemicals in your home or your garage.

• Get an air filter. There are several ways you can filter air. Installing a true HEPA filter with a VOC filter in your furnace will get a lot of the impurities out, including allergens like dust and mold spores. You can also get HEPA filters for your vacuum cleaner. A good-quality air purifier is a great addition, too, especially for the bedrooms; we all spend a lot of time breathing deeply while we sleep. Air purifiers can't filter out everything — for example, they won't remove radon or carbon monoxide — but they definitely help clean out the stuff that could irritate or cause allergies or even asthma in your home.

CLEAN UP YOUR KITCHEN

I'm not talking about your pantry. There are toxins in cleaning products, nonstick cookware, plastics, and more that are hugely detrimental to your health. Fortunately for us, they are fairly easy to eliminate. I want to zero in on the things you use to cook, serve, and store your food in.

Upgrade your cookware: When it comes to what you cook in, be sure to avoid Teflon and all other nonstick pans. The chemicals used to keep foods from sticking are PFAs, or poly- and perfluoroalkyl substances, which have been linked to serious health concerns like infertility, thyroid problems, and even organ damage in animals. At high heat, these synthetic polymers release toxic fumes that can actually kill birds and cause flulike symptoms in humans. Plus, they tend to scratch and flake off into food over time, and although these particles are supposedly inert, those flakes may be made using perfluorooctanoic acid.

Your best option: opt for stainless-steel, cast-iron, ceramic, or glass cookware instead, and just add a little olive oil to keep things from sticking. You'll be all set.

Lose the bleach: Paper towels, paper plates, coffee filters, and napkins—ever wonder how they got so white? These paper products are bleached. Yeah, like with chlorine, which is toxic mostly because when chlorine binds with anything made of carbon (such as paper), it produces extremely harmful dioxins and other pollutants. And although the really toxic bleaching that all paper mills used to employ has largely been replaced by less toxic methods (at least in the United States and Canada), many companies still use chlorine compounds. But why even take a chance?

Your best option: Choose unbleached paper products in your home whenever possible. That means products that use non-chlorine bleaching processes such as oxygen, peroxide, or ozone bleaching methods. The very best choice is processed chlorine-free, or PCF, paper. Products made from PCF paper are chlorine-free and use chlorine-free recycled paper. Put simply, get the brown paper towels and coffee filters instead of the white ones.

Don't worry about your microwave: What was a big concern in the seventies isn't a concern anymore. It's pretty much never been proven that microwaves cause harm to those who use them.

In fact, using a microwave may actually help you age better. Because food takes less time to cook, vitamin C and other nutrients are better preserved, according to Harvard Medical School. The more nutrients you're able to retain in the food you eat, the more protected your body is against aging.

Put thought into your plastics: Never, ever store food in plastic containers, and especially never *heat* food in plastic containers. Plastics are a whole chemical hazard unto themselves; I mentioned this earlier in our 6 Keys chapters, and I discuss it even more extensively in my book *Master Your Metabolism*. Go there if you want all the gory details, but here's the bottom line: some plastics are more dangerous than others, with a few linked to a host of health-related issues like cancer, endocrine disruption, birth defects, and more. But here's a primer. (BTW, to tell which type of plastic you're dealing with, just look for the number stamped somewhere on it.)

Plastics considered unsafe

Polyvinyl chloride (also labeled as V or PVC) — stamped recycle #3: PVC is usually found in cooking-oil bottles; cling wrap; clear wrap around meat, cheese, deli meats, and other food items; plumbing pipes; and toys. This one is truly the worst, both for its environmental impact and for how it accumulates in the human body. Polyvinyl chloride contains hormone disrupters and carcinogens, and both are released into foods when this type of plastic is heated.

Your best option: Choose non-PVC cling wrap, always store food in glass, and buy cooking oil that's kept in glass bottles.

Polystyrene (also labeled as PS) — stamped recycle #6: This type of plastic is found in disposable coffee cups, take-out containers, foam egg cartons, meat trays, packing peanuts, and foam insulation. It's also found in CD jewel cases and in disposable cutlery and transparent take-out containers.

Polystyrenes include benzene, butadiene, and styrene, which are all known or suspected carcinogens, especially when heated. Polystyrene is also an endocrine disruptor. You know those old-school cups of noodles you heat in the microwave? Polystyrene soup, anyone? Or those foam containers you get when ordering take-out? Toxins from these kinds of containers can block the actions and/or disrupt the messages of certain hormones.

Your best option: Never drink hot drinks out of foam cups, eat food from foam containers, or use conventional plastic cutlery on hot foods. Instead, let restaurants know that you care about their take-out containers and bring your business to those that use paper-based take-out containers or containers made from corn or sugar instead of polystyrene. And if you do end up with take-out in a polystyrene container, put it in a glass or ceramic bowl as soon as you get home.

Plastics Considered Possibly Unsafe or Safe — It All Depends

Plastics stamped with recycling category #7 are those that don't fit into the other categories I describe above or below. These plastics can contain anything from dangerous PC (polycarbonate) to harmless PLA (polylactide, a plastic made from corn, potatoes, sugar, or other plant-based starches).

PLAs are awesome because they're 100 persent compostable. Many natural-foods stores and restaurants (and enlightened mainstream stores and restaurants) are switching to these compostable take-out containers. But PC is the bad stuff. It's a polycarbonate plastic that contains bisphenol A (BPA). If you see the letters PC by the number 7, it's the bad stuff. But without those letters, it could be one of thousands of other plastics, and which ones are anybody's guess!

As I've already discussed, some seven hundred studies, mostly on animals, have linked BPA with a host of really, REALLY bad things. It's found in microwave ovenware, stain-resistant food-storage containers, medical storage containers, eating utensils, plastic liners, almost all food and soft-drink cans, Lexan containers, old Nalgene and other hard-plastic water bottles, five-gallon water jugs, building materials, and yes, even baby bottles.

Your best option: Drink from water bottles lined with stainless steel or ceramic and avoid lined aluminum and steel cans, which often contain BPA. Also, never wash BPA-containing plastic in the dishwasher, as this will degrade it further. Once it gets cloudy, throw it away. Common sense note: if you ever smell plastic in any liquid or food, don't drink or eat it!

Plastics Considered Safe — Sort Of

Polyethylene terephthalate (PET or PETE) — stamped recycle #1: This is found in bottles for cough syrup, ketchup, salad dressing, soft drinks, sports drinks, and water. It's also found in plastic jars for pickles, jelly, jam, mustard, mayonnaise, and peanut butter. It's pretty inert, with no known health hazards, and easily recycled into fleece and polyester fabric.

Your best option: Don't re-use water bottles made from this kind of plastic — they can attract bacteria.

High-density polyethylene (HDPE) — stamped recycle #2: It's in toys, shampoo bottles, milk jugs, yogurt containers, margarine tubs, recyclable grocery bags, trash bags, laundry detergent bottles, composite lumber, Tyvek building material, some Tupperware products, sanitary products, original hula hoops, and some shrink wrap. HDPE contains no known endocrine disruptors or carcinogens and is easily recycled.

Your best option: This kind of plastic is fine, as long as you don't microwave food in it, put hot food into it, or leave it out in the sun. Just know that it is made from oil (in an inefficient process), so it's a wasteful product — environmentally speaking.

Low-density polyethylene (LDPE) — stamped recycle #4: You'll find this one in grocery bags, bowls, lids, toys, six-pack rings, trays, power cables, liners, cling wrap, sandwich bags, food coloring and other squeezable bottles, and bottle caps.

Your best option: This is another safe, inert choice, but again, don't warm it up, and know that many recycling centers don't accept this type of plastic. That means when you're done with it, you'll have to throw it away, and it will just end up in landfill.

Polypropylene (PP)—stamped recycle #5: It's commonly used in plastic utensils, cups, thermal underwear (such as Under Armour brand), clear bags, diapers, safe baby bottles, and condiment bottles. This one is not known to be hazardous to those using it, but it can be hazardous to those producing it.

Your best option: It's fine to use, but again, don't heat this one up. It's also not generally accepted at recycling centers.

CREATE A CHEMICAL-FREE YARD

Did you know that 94 percent of households report using some kind of pesticide? And if you hire a landscaper, gardener, pool guy, or exterminator, chances are their tool kit includes some pretty nasty chemicals. Keep your yard clean and pure by avoiding the following:

- Chemical weed killers like Roundup
- Chemical pesticides like Bug Clear, Plant Rescue, Raid Ant Killer
- Chemical fertilizers like Miracle-Gro

Check out www.safelawns.org for tons of useful tips on how to care for your yard, garden, and pool as safely as possible.

CLEAN THINGS THE SMARTEST WAY

You already know that many of the ingredients in standard household cleaning products negatively impact the 6 Keys, causing everything from acute exposure emergencies to long-term hazards like asthma, lung damage, heart damage, and other issues like allergies and headaches. To make matters worse, many contain endocrine disruptors, which interfere with fertility and may cause birth defects and cancer — and that's on top of the horrendous damage they do to the environment.

I'm not going to list all the dangerous chemicals and their effects on the 6 Keys because it would literally take hundreds of pages. Instead, here are my recommendations, along with some DIY solutions to help you green-up your cleanup.

Always look for the following:

- Ammonia-free
- Biodegradable
- Free of dye or perfume
- Noncarcinogenic
- Non-petroleum-based
- Nontoxic

Buy the green brands:

These are brands that I have personally investigated and found to be cleaner, greener, and purer than conventional cleaning products.

- Bona (for hardwood floors)
- Ecover (for dishwasher tablets, laundry detergents, and laundry stain-removing products)
- Honest Company (for laundry detergent, floor cleaners, toilet cleaners, and glass cleaners)
- Method (for furniture polish and toilet cleaners)
- Mrs. Meyer's (for powder surface scrubs and liquid hand soaps)
- Shaklee (for a multi-purpose cleaner)
- Simple Green (for an all-purpose carpet cleaner)
- Skoy (a cloth to replace bleached paper towels and sponges)

Try DIY cleaning products:

There are tons of totally safe products in your own kitchen and bathroom that make excellent cleaners.

- Baking soda (for cleansing and deodorizing)
- Club soda (removes rust and crud from anything and everything)
- Hydrogen peroxide (often used in combination with white vinegar as a sanitizer)
- Lemon juice (serves as a great substitute for bleach)
- Olive oil (an excellent natural furniture and floor polish, plus it gets the fingerprints off stainless-steel appliances)
- Salt (which can do everything from remove stains and mildew to deodorize, and even deter ants)
- Diluted white vinegar (great for cleaning floors, windows, mirrors, and showers; when combined with baking soda, it can even help unclog a sink: just pour in the baking soda, then pour in the vinegar and watch it fizz — kids love it)

GET THE BEST WATER ON TAP

You hopefully drink it all day long, but you also cook with it, bathe in it, and clean with it. Basically, you can't live without it, which is why it's crucial that the water you use is as pollutant-free as possible.

Not all tap water is created equal. Some parts of the United States have excellent tap water and others do not. But here's the thing: municipal water suppliers *must* provide an annual report by July 1 to their customers, and this report provides information on local drinking-water quality, including where your water comes from and what's in it. Those water-quality reports can be obtained by simply contacting suppliers directly or through the EPA's website (www.epa.gov).

But even if your water checks out, I still recommend filters. It's impossible to test for all potential contaminants, even though public water suppliers screen for more than two hundred pollutants. And even if your water is good, your pipes might be leaching chemicals into your tap water. So filter your water. There are many options, but I recommend either installing a reverse osmosis filter or attaching a carbon filter to your faucets.

As for bottled water, the differences among brands are vast. Some brands are literally just tap water in plastic bottles, while others are reverse osmosis purified. Some are alkaline and some have added electrolytes. The list goes on. But if you're going to spend the money, I highly recommend bottled water that is reverse osmosis filtered, alkaline, and enhanced with electrolytes. Personally, I put money into the company Aqua Hydrate and became an investor because it is literally the only brand I can find that has all the above.

PUT YOUR TECH IN CHECK

When it comes to how safe laptops, cell phones, and other electronics are for your 6 Keys, man, this one is tricky because it's an ongoing debate. Why? Because every time something comes out against electronics, the skeptics immediately attempt to debunk it. That said, let's look at what to worry about—and what to wonder about.

Computers: All computers and tablets—all electronics, for that matter—radiate electromagnetic fields (EMF), otherwise known as electromagnetic radiation, which is produced by electrically charged objects. But here's the interesting thing: so does your body. Mind you, it's tiny, but we all give off electromagnetic radiation. But how do you reduce your exposure to excess EMF radiation? The answer is mainly common-sense stuff.

• Stop going wireless for convenience. Wireless devices emit a small radio frequency field, so switching back to a corded mouse, headset, or keyboard could be a safer option, since corded options emit far less radiation.
• Limit your use of computers.
• Move your computer screen as far from you as possible.
• Fill your computer room with plants, since they may help absorb some types of EMF radiation.
• Take your laptop off your lap.
• Stay away from Wi-Fi as much as possible.

I get it, it's a huge pain—especially the Wi-Fi part. That said, the goal with this one is to limit exposure, and every little bit counts when it comes to your 6 Keys.

Smartphones: The cell phone industry is a billion-dollar business. If it's ever definitively proven that cell phones emit radiation that can damage our DNA, just think of how many businesses would be crippled. That news would seriously affect companies such as AT&T, Apple, Verizon, and any social media company, like Facebook or Twitter, where most of its users check their feeds on their phones—and not necessarily on a computer screen.

But let's talk common sense: your cell phone is a two-way radio that does emit a small amount of electromagnetic radiation. And nowadays, who puts their cell phone down? More important, where are you holding it when you're using it? Are you holding it at a safe enough distance, or pressing it to your ear—and right by your brain, I might add—when you talk into it?

It took decades for the truth about cigarettes to finally reach the public, even though common sense should have dictated that inhaling smoke into our lungs wasn't good for us, right? I mean, did we really need hundreds of studies to put two and two together on this one?

That said, if cell phones emit a small amount of electromagnetic radiation, and the debate continues on whether or not that's harmful for us, why not just err on the side of caution and minimize exposure to them as much as possible? Why not keep them at a safe distance as often as you can?

Makes sense, right? Whether that's using a corded headset when speaking on it, holding it as far away from your body as possible when texting, placing it down more often (instead of always having it in your back pocket), whatever. Anything that brings a little distance between you and your phone is a better option than not.

AGE-PROOF YOUR PERSONAL HYGIENE

What you put on your body matters almost as much as what you put in it—and some would say more so. The vast majority of what goes on your body gets absorbed into your body, but it doesn't get filtered by your kidneys or your liver the same way that what you eat and drink does.

You need to be mindful about your hygiene and makeup products. I must admit, it has always surprised me to see women spending hundreds, if not thousands of dollars on beauty products or anti-aging creams that are loaded with toxins that affect the 6 Keys and age them as a result.

In truth, you can totally get away with all-natural ingredients for a fraction of the price, with none of the chemicals, and even a few added health benefits. I use olive oil and coconut oil as moisturizers, and my skin looks and feels great. No chemicals in sight.

If you search online you can find a ton of natural alternatives, from sea-salt and brown-sugar scrubs to hair conditioners using avocados or eggs. But here, let's go over the top offenders that you want to avoid in order to keep your 6 Keys turning in the right direction.

Parabens: These are in about 99 percent of beauty products designed to prevent oxidation and kill bacteria. The problem? They are rapidly absorbed into the skin, accumulate in the body, disrupt critical body processes, and contribute to cancer, metabolic dysfunction, and endocrine disruption.

Where they hide: Watch out for these ingredients—methylparaben, ethylparaben, propylparaben, and butylparaben.

Petrochemicals: Petroleum-based chemicals can be found in mineral oil, petrolatum, and paraffin-based products, even though they (and their by-products) have been linked to serious health problems, including cancer, neuro- and respiratory toxicity, birth defects, and endocrine disruption. They can also cause less serious issues, such as allergic reactions and skin irritation.

Where they hide: Look for the abbreviations PEG (polyethylene glycol), DEA (diethanolamine), MEA (ethanolamine), and SLS (sodium lauryl sulfate), as well as anything with the word *butanol* or *butyl* (such as butyl alcohol or butylene glycol) or *propyl* (such as isopropyl alcohol, propylene glycol, or propyl alcohol).

Fragrance: I know a good fragrance might make you feel sexy or mask bad smells, but it's loaded with petrochemicals, as well as phthalates. Phthalates are endocrine disruptors that mimic hormones and interfere with your normal hormone production.

Where they hide: They sort of don't—you can smell them. Fragrance is in such a wide variety of beauty products, from moisturizers to makeup. If the product lists the words *fragrance, perfume,* or *parfum,* avoid it.

In general, if you seek out natural hygiene and beauty products that don't list any of these words, you're on the right track. But if you don't want to think that hard, look for products that are EWG verified, which means the Environmental Working Group has given them the thumbs-up. Companies earn that EWG verification when their products are free of chemicals believed to be dangerous to human health and the environment, when they disclose all their ingredients, and when they follow good manufacturing practices. To see every hygiene and beauty product that's EWG verified, just go to www.ewg.org/skindeep.

So here's our summary of action steps:

- Clean up your indoor air by looking for and removing/ mitigating the following:
  - Airborne bacteria and viruses
  - Asbestos
  - Carbon monoxide
  - Product off-gassing
  - Mold

- ○ Radon
- ○ Smoke
- ○ Lead
- ○ Any harsh chemicals in your home or garage
- Make a habit of:
  - ○ Opening the windows whenever possible to air out any toxic fumes
  - ○ Investing in house plants
  - ○ Not dry-cleaning your clothes
  - ○ Avoiding air fresheners
  - ○ Investing in air filters (HEPA whenever possible) and cleaning/changing them regularly
- Clean up your kitchen by:
  - ○ Avoiding Teflon and all other nonstick pans and using stainless-steel, cast-iron, ceramic, or glass cookware instead
  - ○ Choosing unbleached paper products
  - ○ Never storing food or *heating up* food in plastic containers, especially if stamped with the numbers 3, 6, or 7
  - ○ Always using non-PVC cling wrap
  - ○ Storing food in glass
  - ○ Only buying cooking oil kept in glass bottles
  - ○ Drinking from water bottles lined with stainless steel or ceramic
- Clean up your yard by avoiding the use of chemical weed killers, pesticides, and fertilizers.
- Clean your things with the following types of products:
  - ○ Ammonia-free
  - ○ Biodegradable
  - ○ Free of dye or perfume
  - ○ Noncarcinogenic

- ○ Non–petroleum-based
- ○ Nontoxic
- Consider using DIY cleaning products such as baking soda, club soda, hydrogen peroxide, lemon juice, olive oil, salt, and diluted white vinegar.
- Check the quality of your drinking water and opt for filtered water as often as possible.
- Minimize your exposure to EMFs by:
  - ○ Switching to a corded mouse, headset, or keyboard instead of going wireless
  - ○ Limiting your use of computers, never putting your laptop in your lap, and filling your computer room with plants
  - ○ Moving your smartphone and/or computer screen as far from you as possible
  - ○ Staying away from Wi-Fi as much as possible
- Avoid any personal hygiene products that contain parabens, petrochemicals, or fragrances.

Conclusion

It's a lot to take in.

I get it. And ultimately, if you get overwhelmed and decide you want a little extra handholding you can try out the 6 Keys diet and fitness program within the My Fitness App: https://www.jillianmichaels.com/6keys2app.

But over time, it will become easier and easier until it's relatively second nature. And as you begin to notice the changes within yourself, I promise that you will be even more inspired to stay the course. Your waistline will slim down, your body will be firmer, your skin will look brighter, your hair will be thicker, you'll have more energy, you'll get sick less often—you'll age well. With grace and beauty, inside and out.

Honestly, it's gonna be awesome.

And while immortality is still out of reach and death is inevitable, I want you to have an incredible time while you're here and make the absolute most of it—or what's it all for, anyway? Find meaning in your life, pursue joy, learn from failures, and grow from losses. And follow the path I've laid out for you here.

Laugh at every opportunity, cry when you feel the need, learn to tango, sing often, and, when love calls, follow it—no matter how much you may fear it. And if your heart breaks, mend it. Per Hemingway, "The world breaks everyone and afterward many are strong at the broken places." Point being: I want you to be stronger in the places your heart has broken—but not harder.

Skinny dip (at least once), have sex, have . . . fun. Sleep. Whenever and wherever you can. Just crash out. Be the person on the subway with a little drool in the corner of your mouth that people snap cell phone pics of. But the joke's on them, cause you're gonna stay hot as f*@# and your telomeres will be way longer.

If you don't like where you're at, move. You're not a mountain. Don't read, watch, or listen to things that make you feel bad about yourself, and don't date a-holes, because you're wonderful and totally worthy of being loved. You really are.

Follow the middle path and avoid extremes of any kind. Anything with the word *too* in front of it is not good.

Eat well—not too much and not too little. Enjoy a glass of wine, have a cup of coffee, and eat that square of dark chocolate. But don't drive into the drive-through and eat fast food. If you're gonna say f*ck it when it comes to food, then do it for something ridiculous like kombucha and chia pudding—not the ten-pound-patty burger with extra sauce and extra cheese.

Exercise like your life depends on it—because it does. Complete a 5K. Accomplish five pull-ups. Climb the Empire State Building. And get a dog. Then, maybe exercise *with* the dog.

Brush your teeth . . . for the full two minutes. And floss. Then get a little crazy with those DIY honey, yogurt, avocado charcoal scrubs, masks, and moisturizers.

Smell the roses, and if you don't like roses, f*ck 'em. Just pick another flower and smell that. Take your vacations. Visit Stonehenge, ride a gondola in Venice, or hike the Great Wall of China.

Remove toxicity from your life, whether it's your mascara or your crappy boss—even if it takes you a while to formulate an exit strategy.

If you have kids, hug them—every chance you get. Put your phone down when they walk into the room and tell them you love them, even if they're on their own phones. Call your parents, so when the day comes that you can't, you'll have that many more memories to look back on.

Create space for quiet time and breathing. Find forgiveness, and if you want to give up on something, make it worrying. (That shit's about as effective a problem-solving skill as brushing your hair—with the brush on fire.)

Be kind. Not because you're anxious about karma or retribution, but because it feels better than being a dick.

Finally, remember that the rat race really only has a party of one...you.

So, slow down.

Truly *take your time*—because it's your most precious commodity. Reach out and grab that sh*t with both hands. Bend it to your will where you can, but don't waste time trying to push the river—roll with it and enjoy the ride.

Acknowledgments

A giant thanks to everyone who helped make this book the go-to manual for being your best self and a smashing manifesto on how to live your best life.

To my book agent, Heather Jackson. Thank you for always being my rock no matter what role you play in my life.

My uber-talented coauthor, Myatt Murphy. Hope your family forgives me for keeping you up all those late nights poring over study after study together.

Tracy Behar and the whole team at Little, Brown: appreciate all your hard work and expertise.

And to my business partner, Giancarlo Chersich, and my whole team at Empowered Media: Sarah, Julie, Kenneth, Cathleen, July, Julia, Eric, Dan, and Haley. Your tireless dedication and commitment make it possible for me to do what I do and for all of us to help others achieve their goals and dreams of health and happiness.

Notes

Chapter 1. Which Age Defines You?

1. Christopher Lee and Myra Fernandes, "Emotional Encoding Context Leads to Memory Bias in Individuals with High Anxiety," *Brain Sciences* 8 (December 2017): 6, doi:10.3390/brainsci8010006.
2. Ramzan Shahid, Jerold Stirling, and William Adams, "Assessment of Emotional Intelligence in Pediatric and Med-Peds Residents," *Journal of Contemporary Medical Education* 4 (2017): 153, doi:10.5455/jcme.20170116015415.
3. Denise Aydinonat et al., "Social Isolation Shortens Telomeres in African Grey Parrots (*Psittacus erithacus erithacus*)," *PLoS ONE* 9(4) (2014): e93839, doi:10.1371/journal.pone.0093839.
4. T. Larrieu et al., "Hierarchical status predicts behavioral vulnerability and nucleus accumbens metabolic profile following chronic social defeat stress," *Current Biology* (July 2017): doi:10.1016/j.cub.2017.06.027.
5. Chris Segrin, "Indirect Effects of Social Skills on Health Through Stress and Loneliness," *Health Communication* (2017): 1, doi:10.1080/10410236.2017.1384434.
6. B. S. Diniz et al., "Plasma biosignature and brain pathology related to persistent cognitive impairment in late-life depression," *Molecular Psychiatry* (2014): doi:10.1038/mp.2014.76.
7. Endocrine Society, "Declining testosterone levels in men not part of normal aging," *ScienceDaily* 23 (June 2012).
8. Mikael Wikgren et al., "Short Telomeres in Depression and the General Population Are Associated with a Hypocortisolemic State," *Biological Psychiatry* (2011): doi:10.1016/j.biopsych.2011.09.015.
9. Jennifer A. Bellingtier and Shevaun D. Neupert, "Negative Aging Attitudes Predict Greater Reactivity to Daily Stressors in Older Adults," *Journal of Gerontology: Psychological Sciences* (August 2016).
10. Deirdre A. Robertson and Rose Anne Kenny, "Negative perceptions of aging modify the association between frailty and cognitive function in older adults," *Personality and Individual Differences* (2015).
11. Michael Greenwood, "Negative beliefs about aging predict Alzheimer's disease in Yale-led study," YaleNews (December 2015): http://news.yale

.edu/2015/12/07/negative-beliefs-about-aging-predict-alzheimer-s
-disease-yale-led-study.

Chapter 2. The Truth About Aging

1. A. M. Berzlanovich et al., "Do centenarians die healthy? An autopsy study," *The Journals of Gerontology, Series A Biological and Medical Sciences* 60, no. 7 (2005): 862–865.
2. Z. A. Medvedev, "An attempt at a rational classification of theories of ageing," *Biology Review* 65 (1990): 375–398.

Chapter 3. The 6 Keys to Unlock Longevity and Vitality

1. J. A. Mattison et al., "Caloric restriction improves health and survival of rhesus monkeys," *Nature Communications* 8 (2017): 14063, doi:10.1038/ncomms14063.
2. C. López-Otín et al., "The Hallmarks of Aging," *Cell* 153, no. 6 (2013): 1194–1217, doi:10.1016/j.cell.2013.05.039.
3. B. K. Kennedy, "Geroscience: linking aging to chronic disease," Cell 159, no. 4 (November 2014): 709–13, doi:10.1016/j.cell.2014.10.039.

Chapter 4. The First Key: Mastering Macromolecules

1. A. G. Richardson and E.E. Schadt, "The role of macromolecular damage in aging and age-related disease," *The Journals of Gerontology, Series A Biological and Medical Sciences* 69 (June 2014): S28–32, doi:10.1093/gerona/glu056.
2. Tamara Tchkonia et al., "Cellular Senescence and the Senescent Secretory Phenotype: Therapeutic Opportunities," *Journal of Clinical Investigation* 123, no. 3 (March 1, 2013): 966–72, doi:10.1172/JCI64098.
3. Michael T. Ryan and Nicholas J. Hoogenraad, "Mitochondrial-Nuclear Communications," *Annual Review of Biochemistry* 76 (2007): 701–22, doi:10.1146/annurev.biochem.76.052305.091720.
4. G. Kroemer, L. Galluzzi, and C. Brenner, "Mitochondrial membrane permeabilization in cell death," Physiology Review 87, no. 1 (January 2007): 99–163.
5. Ryan Doonan et al., "Against the Oxidative Damage Theory of Aging: Superoxide Dismutases Protect against Oxidative Stress but Have Little or No Effect on Life Span in *Caenorhabditis Elegans*," *Genes & Development* 22, no. 23 (December 1, 2008): 3236–41, doi:10.1101/gad.504808.
6. Susmita Kaushik and Ana Maria Cuervo, "Proteostasis and Aging," *Nature Medicine* 21, no. 12 (December 2015): 1406–15, doi:10.1038/nm.4001.
7. J. A. Carver et al., "Proteostasis and the Regulation of Intra- and Extracellular Protein Aggregation by ATP-Independent Molecular Chaperones: Lens α-Crystallins and Milk Caseins," *Accounts of Chemical Research* 51, no. 3 (March 2018): 745–52, doi:10.1021/acs.accounts.7b00250.

J. F. Díaz-Villanueva, R. Díaz-Molina, and V. García-González, "Protein Folding and Mechanisms of Proteostasis," *International Journal of Molecular Sciences,* S. Ventura (ed.), 16, no. 8 (2015): 17193-17230, doi:10.3390/ijms160817193.

Robert H. Henning and Bianca J. J. Brundel, "Proteostasis in cardiac health and disease," *Nature Reviews Cardiology* 14, no. 11 (November 2017): 637–53, doi:10.1038/nrcardio.2017.89.

P. M. Douglas and A. Dillin, "Protein homeostasis and aging in neurodegeneration," *The Journal of Cell Biology* 190, no. 5 (2010): 719–29, doi:10.1083/jcb.201005144.

8. M. Murga, et al., "A mouse model of ATR-Seckel shows embryonic replicative stress and accelerated aging," *Nature Genetics* 41 (2009): 891–98.

9. A. A. Freitas and J. P. Magalhães, "A review and appraisal of the DNA damage theory of ageing," *Mutation Research* 728, nos. 1–2 (July–October 2011): 12–22, doi:10.1016/j.mrrev.2011.05.001.

10. Celia Pilar Martinez-Jimenez et al., "Aging increases cell-to-cell transcriptional variability upon immune stimulation," *Science* 355, no. 6332 (2017): 1433.

11. Sam Palmer et al., "Thymic involution and rising disease incidence with age," *PNAS* (2018), doi:10.1073/pnas.1714478115.

12. The Endocrine Society, "Stem cell therapy may help reverse effects of premature menopause, restore fertility," *ScienceDaily* 18 (March 2018).

13. Lyndon da Cruz et al., "Phase 1 clinical study of an embryonic stem cell–derived retinal pigment epithelium patch in age-related macular degeneration," *Nature Biotechnology* (2018): doi:10.1038/nbt.4114.

14. Peng Liu et al., "CRISPR-Based Chromatin Remodeling of the Endogenous Oct4 or Sox2 Locus Enables Reprogramming to Pluripotency," *Cell Stem Cell* (2018): doi:10.1016/j.stem.2017.12.001.

15. https://stemcells.nih.gov/info/basics/7.htm.

16. M. Conese et al., (2017). "The Fountain of Youth: A tale of parabiosis, stem cells, and rejuvenation," *Open Medicine* 12, no. 1 (2017): 376–83.

17. M. Sinha, "Restoring systemic GDF11 levels reverses age-related dysfunction in mouse skeletal muscle," *Science* 344, no. 6184 (May 2014): 649–52, doi:10.1126/science.1251152.

18. J. M. Castellano, "Human umbilical cord plasma proteins revitalize hippocampal function in aged mice," *Nature* 544, no. 7651 (April 2017): 488–92.

19. Bruno Bernardes de Jesus et al., "Silencing of the lncRNA Zeb2-NAT facilitates reprogramming of aged fibroblasts and safeguards stem cell pluripotency," *Nature Communications* 9, no. 1 (2018): doi:10.1038/s41467-017-01921-6

20. Junichi Taniguchi et al., "A synthetic DNA-binding inhibitor of SOX2 guides human induced pluripotent stem cells to differentiate into

mesoderm," *Nucleic Acids Research* 45, no. 16 (2017): 9219, doi:10.1093/nar/gkx693.

21. Jun Li et al., "A conserved NAD binding pocket that regulates protein-protein interactions during aging," *Science* 355, no. 6331 (March 2017): 1312–17.

22. Eva Latorre et al., "Small molecule modulation of splicing factor expression is associated with rescue from cellular senescence," *BMC Cell Biology* 18, no. 1 (2017): doi:10.1186/s12860-017-0147-7.

23. Samantha Haller et al., "mTORC1 Activation during Repeated Regeneration Impairs Somatic Stem Cell Maintenance," *Cell Stem Cell* 21, no. 6 (2017): 806, doi:10.1016/j.stem.2017.11.008.

24. B. Onken and M. Driscoll, "Metformin induces a dietary restriction-like state and the oxidative stress response to extend *C. elegans* Healthspan via AMPK, LKB1, and SKN-1," *PLoS ONE* 5 (2010): e8758.

    V. N. Anisimov et al., "If started early in life, metformin treatment increases life span and postpones tumors in female SHR mice," *Aging* 3 (2011): 148–57.

25. Yalin Zhang et al., "Hypothalamic stem cells control aging speed partly through exosomal miRNAs," *Nature* (2017): doi:10.1038/nature23282.

26. X. Zhang et al., "MCOLN1 is a ROS sensor in lysosomes that regulates autophagy," *Nature Communications* 7 (June 2016): 12109.

27. Mark Y. Jeng et al., "Metabolic reprogramming of human CD8 memory T cells through loss of SIRT1," *The Journal of Experimental Medicine* (2017): jem.20161066, doi:10.1084/jem.20161066.

28. C. Correia-Melo et al., "Mitochondria are required for pro-ageing features of the senescent phenotype," *EMBO* 35, no. 7 (April 2016): 724-42, doi:10.15252/embj.201592862.

29. Maria M. Mihaylova et al., "Fasting Activates Fatty Acid Oxidation to Enhance Intestinal Stem Cell Function during Homeostasis and Aging," *Cell Stem Cell* 22, no. 5 (2018): 769.

30. N. L. Bodkin et al., "Mortality and morbidity in laboratory-maintained Rhesus monkeys and effects of long-term dietary restriction." *The Journals of Gerontology, Series A Biological and Medical Sciences* 58, no. 3 (2003): 212–19.

31. D. Il'yasova et al., "Effects of 2 years of caloric restriction on oxidative status assessed by urinary F2-isoprostanes: The CALERIE 2 randomized clinical trial," *Aging Cell* 17, no. 2 (April 2018): doi:10.1111/acel.12719.

32. A. E. Civitarese et al., "Calorie restriction increases muscle mitochondrial biogenesis in healthy humans," *PLoS Medicine* 4, no. 3 (March 2007): e76.

    T. Hofer et al., "Long-term effects of caloric restriction or exercise on DNA and RNA oxidation levels in white blood cells and urine in humans," *Rejuvenation Research* 11 (2008): 793–99.

    M. Lefevre et al., "Caloric restriction alone and with exercise improves CVD risk in healthy non–obese individuals," *Atherosclerosis* 203 (2009): 206–13.

33. L. O. Dragsted et al., "The 6-a-day study: effects of fruit and vegetables on markers of oxidative stress and antioxidative defense in healthy nonsmokers," *American Journal of Clinical Nutrition* 79, no. 6 (June 2004): 1060–72.

34. Sangyong Choi et al., "Selective inhibitory effects of zinc on cell proliferation in esophageal squamous cell carcinoma through Orai1, *The FASEB Journal* (2017): fj.201700227RRR, doi:10.1096/fj.201700227RRR.

35. Janice K. Kiecolt-Glaser, Martha A. Belury, Rebecca Andridge, William B. Malarkey, Beom Seuk Hwang, Ronald Glaser, "Omega-3 supplementation lowers inflammation in healthy middle-aged and older adults: A randomized controlled trial," *Brain, Behavior, and Immunity*, 2012; 26 (6): 988:

36. Luisa Cimmino et al., "Restoration of TET2 Function Blocks Aberrant Self-Renewal and Leukemia Progression," *Cell* (2017): doi:10.1016/j. cell.2017.07.032.

37. T. Ramani et al., "Cytokines: The Good, the Bad, and the Deadly," *International Journal of Toxicology* 34, no. 4 (July–August 2015): 355–65, doi:10.1177/ 1091581815584918.

38. T. A. Lennie, "Dietary fat intake and proinflammatory cytokine levels in patients with heart failure," *Journal of Cardiac Failure* 11, no. 8 (October 2005): 613–18.

39. J. Urinbarri et al., "Dietary advanced glycation end products and their role in health and disease," *Advances in Nutrition* 6, no. 4 (July 2015): 461–73, doi:10.3945/an.115.008433.

40. McGill University Health Centre, "Eating protein three times a day could make our seniors stronger: Quebec researchers link protein distribution to greater mass and muscle strength in the elderly," *ScienceDaily*, www.science daily.com/releases/2017/08/170830202131.htm.

41. P. Boor et al., "Regular moderate exercise reduces advanced glycation and ameliorates early diabetic nephropathy in obese Zucker rats," *Metabolism* 58, no. 11 (November 2009): 1669–77, doi:10.1016/j.metabol.2009 .05.025.

    J. P. Little et al., "Low-volume high-intensity interval training reduces hyperglycemia and increases muscle mitochondrial capacity in patients with type 2 diabetes," *Journal of Applied Physiology* 111, no. 6 (December 2011): 1554–60, doi:10.1152/japplphysiol.00921.2011.

    A. Safdar et al., "Endurance exercise rescues progeroid aging and induces systemic mitochondrial rejuvenation in mtDNA mutator mice," *PNAS* 108, no. 10 (March 2011): 4135–40, doi:10.1073/pnas.1019581108.

42. Matthew M. Robinson et al., "Enhanced Protein Translation Underlies Improved Metabolic and Physical Adaptations to Different Exercise Training Modes in Young and Old Humans," *Cell Metabolism* 25, no. 3 (2017): 581.

43. M. C. Gomez-Cabrera, E. Domenech, and J. Viña, "Moderate exercise is an antioxidant: upregulation of antioxidant genes by training," *Free Radical*

Biology and Medicine 44, no. 2 (January 2008): 126–31, doi:10.1016/j. freeradbiomed.2007.02.001.

44. Harshavardhan Kenche et al., "Adverse Outcomes Associated with Cigarette Smoke Radicals Related to Damage to Protein-disulfide Isomerase," *Journal of Biological Chemistry* 291, no. 9 (2016): 4763.

45. American Academy of Sleep Medicine, "Partial sleep deprivation linked to biological aging in older adults," *ScienceDaily* (June 2015).

46. Yasmine M. Cissé, Kathryn L.G. Russart, and Randy J. Nelson, "Parental Exposure to Dim Light at Night Prior to Mating Alters Offspring Adaptive Immunity," *Scientific Reports* 7 (2017): 45497.

Chapter 5. The Second Key: Engineering Epigenetics

1. A. Zykovich et al., "Genome-wide DNA methylation changes with age in disease-free human skeletal muscle," *Aging Cell* 13, no. 2 (2014): 360–66.

   Christoph D. Rau and Thomas M. Vondriska, "DNA Methylation and Human Heart Failure," *Circulation* 136 (2017): 1545–47, originally published October 16, 2017.

   S. Zaina et al., "DNA methylation map of human atherosclerosis," *Circulation: Cardiovascular Genetics* 7, no. 5 (2014): 692–700.

2. S. B. Baylin and P. A. Jones, "A decade of exploring the cancer epigenome — biological and translational implications," *Nature Reviews Cancer* 11, no. 10 (2011): 726–34.

3. M. J. Hoffmann and W. A. Schulz, "Causes and consequences of DNA hypomethylation in human cancer," *Biochemistry and Cell Biology* 83, no. 3 (2005): 296–321.

   A. Zykovich et al., "Genome-wide DNA methylation changes with age in disease-free human skeletal muscle," *Aging Cell* 13, no. 2 (2014): 360–66.

   D. A. Bennett et al., "Epigenomics of Alzheimer's disease," *Translational Research* 165, no. 1 (2015): 200–20.

4. Z. Xu and J. A. Taylor, "Genome-wide age-related DNA methylation changes in blood and other tissues relate to histone modification, expression and cancer," *Carcinogenesis* 35, no. 2 (2014): 356–64.

5. S. Peleg et al., "Life span extension by targeting a link between metabolism and histone acetylation in *Drosophila, EMBO Reports* 17, no. 3 (March 2016: 455–69, doi:10.15252/embr.201541132.

6. F. Zenk et al., "Germ line-inherited H3K27me3 restricts enhancer function during maternal-to-zygotic transition," *Science* 357, no. 6347 (July 2017): 212–16, doi:10.1126/science.aam5339.

7. Richard Pilsner et al., "Preconception urinary phthalate concentrations and sperm DNA methylation profiles among men undergoing IVF treatment: a cross-sectional study," *Human Reproduction* (September 2017): doi:10.1093/humrep/dex283.

8. M. V. Veenendaal et al., "Transgenerational effects of prenatal exposure to the 1944–45 Dutch famine," *BJOG* 120, no. 5 (April 2013): 548–53, doi:10.1111/1471-0528.12136.

9. Elizabeth M. Curtis et al., "Perinatal DNA methylation at CDKN2A is associated with offspring bone mass: Findings from the Southampton Women's Survey," *Journal of Bone and Mineral Research* (2017): doi:10.1002/jbmr.3153.

10. Jihoon E. Joo et al., "Heritable DNA methylation marks associated with susceptibility to breast cancer," *Nature Communications* 9, no. 1 (2018): doi:10.1038/s41467-018-03058-6.

11. Rachel Yehuda et al., "Holocaust exposure induced intergenerational effects on *FKBP5* methylation," *Biological Psychiatry* 80, no. 5 (September 2016): 372–380.

12. Adam Klosin et al., "Transgenerational transmission of environmental information in *C. elegans*," Science 356, no. 6335 (April 2017): 320–23.

13. https://cancergenome.nih.gov/abouttcga/overview.

14. E. S. Lander, "The Heroes of CRISPR," Cell 164, no. 1–2 (January 2016): 18–28, doi:10.1016/j.cell.2015.12.041.

15. E. Lin-Shiao et al., "KMT2D regulates p63 target enhancers to coordinate epithelial homeostasis," *Genes & Development* 32, no. 2 (2018): 181–93.

16. G. Vogt et al., "Production of different phenotypes from the same genotype in the same environment by developmental variation," *Journal of Experimental Biology* 211, no. 4 (February 2008): 510–23, doi:10.1242/jeb.008755.

17. Shinji Maegawa et al., "Caloric restriction delays age-related methylation drift," *Nature Communications* 8, no. 1 (2017): doi:10.1038/s41467-017-00607-3.

18. K. Szarc vel Szic et al., "From inflammaging to healthy aging by dietary lifestyle choices: is epigenetics the key to personalized nutrition?" *Clinical Epigenetics* 7, no. 1 (2015): 33.

19. S. C. Jacobsen et al., "Effects of short-term high-fat overfeeding on genome-wide DNA methylation in the skeletal muscle of healthy young men," *Diabetologia* 55, no. 12 (December 2012): 3341–9, doi:10.1007/s00125-012-2717-8.

20. R. A. J. Zwamborn et al., "Prolonged high-fat diet induces gradual and fat depot-specific DNA methylation changes in adult mice," *Scientific Reports* 7 (2017): 43261, doi:10.1038/srep43261.

21. E. C. Yiannakopoulou, "Targeting DNA methylation with green tea catechins," *Pharmacology* 95, no. 3–4 (2015): 111–6, doi:10.1159/000375503.

22. A. Giudice et al., "Epigenetic Changes Induced by Green Tea Catechins are Associated with Prostate Cancer," *Current Molecular Medicine* 17, no. 6 (2017): 405–20, doi:10.2174/1566524018666171219101937.

23. K. S. Crider et al., " Folate and DNA Methylation: A Review of Molecular Mechanisms and the Evidence for Folate's Role," *Advances in Nutrition* 3, no. 1 (2012): 21–38, doi:10.3945/an.111.000992.

24. Yiting Zhang et al., "Decreased Brain Levels of Vitamin B12 in Aging, Autism and Schizophrenia," *PLOS One* 11, no. 1 (2016): e0146797, doi:10.1371/journal.pone.0146797.

25. S. Reuter et al., "Epigenetic changes induced by curcumin and other natural compounds," *Genes & Nutrition* 6, no. 2 (2011): 93–108, doi:10.1007/s12263-011-0222-1.

26. Sarandeep S. S. Boyanapalli and Ah-Ng Tony Kong, "'Curcumin, the King of Spices': Epigenetic Regulatory Mechanisms in the Prevention of Cancer, Neurological, and Inflammatory Diseases," *Current Pharmacology Reports* 1, no. 2 (2015): 129–39, doi:10.1007/s40495-015-0018-x.

27. M. E. Lindholm et al., "An integrative analysis reveals coordinated reprogramming of the epigenome and the transcriptome in human skeletal muscle after training," *Epigenetics* 9, no. 12 (December 2014): 1557–69, doi: 10.4161/15592294.2014.982445.

28. Robert A. Seaborne et al., "Human Skeletal Muscle Possesses an Epigenetic Memory of Hypertrophy," *Scientific Reports* 8, no. 1 (2018): doi:10.1038/s41598-018-20287-3.

29. Tina Rönn et al., "A Six Months Exercise Intervention Influences the Genome-wide DNA Methylation Pattern in Human Adipose Tissue," *PLoS Genetics* 9, no. 6 (2013): e1003572, doi:10.1371/journal.pgen.1003572.

30. M. Hamer, K. L. Lavoie, and S. L. Bacon, "Taking up physical activity in later life and healthy ageing: the English longitudinal study of ageing," *British Journal of Sports Medicine* 48 (2013): 239–243.

31. W. M. Brown, "Exercise-associated DNA methylation change in skeletal muscle and the importance of imprinted genes: a bioinformatics meta-analysis," *British Journal of Sports Medicine* 49, no. 24 (2015): 1567–78.

32. Simone Wahl et al., "Epigenome-wide association study of body mass index, and the adverse outcomes of adiposity," *Nature* (2016): doi:10.1038/nature20784.

33. Roby Joehanes et al., "Epigenetic Signatures of Cigarette Smoking," *Circulation: Cardiovascular Genetics* (2016): doi:10.1161/CIRCGENETICS.116.001506.

34. L. Tan et al., "Bisphenol A exposure accelerated the aging process in the nematode *Caenorhabditis elegans*," *Toxicology Letters* 235, no. 1 (June 2015): 75–83, doi:10.1016/j.toxlet.2015.03.010.

35. M. Manikkam et al., "Transgenerational actions of environmental compounds on reproductive disease and identification of epigenetic biomarkers of ancestral exposures," *PLoS One* 7 (2012): e31901.

36. S. Singh and S. S. L. Li, "Epigenetic Effects of Environmental Chemicals Bisphenol A and Phthalates," *International Journal of Molecular Sciences* 13, no. 8 (2012): 10143–53, doi:10.3390/ijms130810143.

37. Kyoung-Nam Kim et al., "Association between phthalate exposure and lower handgrip strength in an elderly population," *Environmental Health,* 2016 15:93.

38. A. J. Cruz-Jentoft et al., "Sarcopenia: European consensus on definition and diagnosis: Report of the European Working Group on Sarcopenia in Older People," *Age and Ageing* 39 (2010): 412–23.

39. M. Gallucci et al., "Body mass index, lifestyles, physical performance and cognitive decline: the 'Treviso Longeva (TRELONG)' study," *Journal of Nutrition, Health and Aging* 17 (2013): 378–84.

   C. H. Hirsch et al., "Predicting late-life disability and death by the rate of decline in physical performance measures," *Age and Ageing* 41 (2012): 155–61.

   M. C. Buser, H. E. Murray, and F. Scinicariello, "Age and sex differences in childhood and adulthood obesity association with phthalates: analyses of NHANES 2007–2010," *International Journal of Hygiene and Environmental Health* 217 (2014): 687–94.

40. J. Holt-Lunstad et al., "Loneliness and Social Isolation as Risk Factors for Mortality: A Meta-Analytic Review," *Perspectives on Psychological Science* 10, no. 2 (2015): 227, doi:10.1177/1745691614568352.

41. B. W. Haas et al., "Epigenetic modification of OXT and human sociability," *PNAS* 113, no. 27 (July 2016): E3816–23, doi:10.1073/pnas.1602809113.

42. Sarah R. Moore et al., "Epigenetic correlates of neonatal contact in humans," *Development and Psychopathology* 29, no. 5 (2017): 1517, doi:10.1017/S0954579417001213.

Chapter 6. The Third Key: Strong-Arming Stress

1. E. S. Epel and G. J. Lithgow, "Stress Biology and Aging Mechanisms: Toward Understanding the Deep Connection Between Adaptation to Stress and Longevity," *Journals of Gerontology Series A: Biological Sciences and Medical Sciences* 69, no. 1 (2014): S10–S16, doi:10.1093/gerona/glu055.

2. Michael D. Nissen, Erica K. Sloan, and Stephen R. Mattarollo, "Beta-adrenergic signaling impairs anti-tumor CD8 T cell responses to B cell lymphoma immunotherapy," *Cancer Immunology Research* (2017): doi:10.1158/2326-6066.CIR-17-0401.

3. Martin Picard and Bruce S. McEwen, "Psychological Stress and Mitochondria," *Psychosomatic Medicine* 80, no. 2 (2018): 141, doi:10.1097/PSY.0000000000000545.

4. S. Rangaraju et al., "Stress and Longevity: Convergence on ANK3," *Molecular Psychiatry* (May 2016).

5. Zahra Bahrami-Nejad et al., "A Transcriptional Circuit Filters Oscillating Circadian Hormonal Inputs to Regulate Fat Cell Differentiation," *Cell Metabolism* 27, no. 4 (2018): 854, doi:10.1016/j.cmet.2018.03.012.

6. J. K. Kiecolt-Glaser et al., "Daily stressors, past depression, and metabolic responses to high-fat meals: a novel path to obesity," *Biological Psychiatry* 77, no. 7 (April 2015): 653–60, doi:10.1016/j.biopsych.2014.05.018.

7. Laura C. Bridgewater et al., "Gender-based differences in host behavior and gut microbiota composition in response to high fat diet and stress in a mouse model," *Scientific Reports* 7, no. 1 (2017): doi:10.1038/s41598-017-11069-4.

8. A. A. Prather et al., "Longevity factor klotho and chronic psychological stress," *Translational Psychiatry* 5, no. 6 (June 2015): e585.

9. Duraisamy Kempuraj et al., "Mast Cell Activation in Brain Injury, Stress, and Post-traumatic Stress Disorder and Alzheimer's Disease Pathogenesis," *Frontiers in Neuroscience* 11.

10. S. I. Rattan, "Hormesis in aging," *Ageing Research Reviews* 7, no. 1 (January 2008): 63–78.

11. Johnathan Labbadia et al., "Mitochondrial Stress Restores the Heat Shock Response and Prevents Proteostasis Collapse during Aging," *Cell Reports* 21, no. 6 (2017): 1481, doi:10.1016/j.celrep.2017.10.038.

12. M. F. Dallman et al., "Chronic stress and obesity: a new view of 'comfort food," *PNAS* 100 (2003): 11696–11701.

13. A. Kokavec et al., "Ingesting alcohol prior to food can alter the activity of the hypothalamic-pituitary-adrenal axis," *Pharmacology Biochemistry and Behavior* 93, no. 2 (2009): 170–6, doi:10.1016/j.pbb.2009.05.004.

14. S. K. Blaine et al., "Alcohol Effects on Stress Pathways: Impact on Craving and Relapse Risk," *Canadian Journal of Psychiatry Revue* 61, no. 3 (2016): 145–153, doi:10.1177/0706743716632512.

15. K. Wunsch, N. Kasten, and R. Fuchs, "The effect of physical activity on sleep quality, well-being, and affect in academic stress periods," *Nature and Science of Sleep* 9 (2017): 117–126, doi:10.2147/NSS.S132078.

16. Roxanne M. Miller et al., "Running exercise mitigates the negative consequences of chronic stress on dorsal hippocampal long-term potentiation in male mice," *Neurobiology of Learning and Memory* 149 (2018): 28, doi:10.1016/j.nlm.2018.01.008.

17. Ivana Buric et al., "What Is the Molecular Signature of Mind–Body Interventions? A Systematic Review of Gene Expression Changes Induced by Meditation and Related Practices," *Frontiers in Immunology* 8 (2017).

18. American Physiological Society, "Stress hormones spike as the temperature rises: Study surprisingly finds higher cortisol levels in summer than in winter," *ScienceDaily*, https://www.sciencedaily.com/releases/2018/04/180425131906.htm (accessed June 5, 2018).

Chapter 7. The Fourth Key: Owning Inflammation

1. Shruti Naik et al., "Inflammatory memory sensitizes skin epithelial stem cells to tissue damage," *Nature* (2017), doi:10.1038/nature24271.

2. Y. Arai et al., "Inflammation, But Not Telomere Length, Predicts Successful Ageing at Extreme Old Age: A Longitudinal Study of Semi-supercentenarians," *EBioMedicine* 2, no. 10 (July 2015): 1549–58.

3. C. Franceschi and J. Campisi, "Chronic inflammation (inflammaging) and its potential contribution to age-associated diseases," *Journals of Gerontology* 69 (2014): S4–9.

4. S. I. Grivennikov, F. R. Greten, and M. Karin, "Immunity, Inflammation, and Cancer," *Cell* 140, no. 6 (2010): 883–899.

5. J. Doles et al., "Age-associated inflammation inhibits epidermal stem cell function," *Genes & Development* 26, no. 19 (October 2012): 2144–53.

6. Britta Wåhlin-Larsson et al., "Mechanistic Links Underlying the Impact of C-Reactive Protein on Muscle Mass in Elderly," *Cellular Physiology and Biochemistry* 267 (2017), doi:10.1159/000484679.

7. Eric M. Pietras et al., "Chronic interleukin-1 exposure drives haematopoietic stem cells towards precocious myeloid differentiation at the expense of self-renewal," *Nature Cell Biology* (2016), doi:10.1038/ncb3346.

8. Keenan A. Walker et al., "Midlife systemic inflammatory markers are associated with late-life brain volume," *Neurology* (2017), doi:10.1212/WNL .0000000000004688.

9. Y. Tang and D. Cai, "Hypothalamic inflammation and GnRH in aging development," *Cell Cycle* 12, no. 17 (2013): 2711–2712, doi:10.4161/cc.26054.

10. G. Zhang et al., "Hypothalamic Programming of Systemic Aging Involving IKKβ/NF-κB and GnRH," *Nature* 497, no. 7448 (2013): 211–216, doi:10.1038/nature12143.

11. Remi-Martin Laberge et al., "MTOR regulates the pro-tumorigenic senescence-associated secretory phenotype by promoting IL1A translation," *Nature Cell Biology* (2015): doi:10.1038/ncb3195.

12. P. M. Ridker et al., "Antiinflammatory Therapy with Canakinumab for Atherosclerotic Disease," *New England Journal of Medicine* 377, no. 12 (September 2017): 1119–1131.

R. A. Harrington, "Targeting Inflammation in Coronary Artery Disease," *New England Journal of Medicine* 377, no. 12 (September 2017): 1197–1198.

13. Xianyi Meng et al., "Hypoxia-inducible factor-1α is a critical transcription factor for IL-10-producing B cells in autoimmune disease," *Nature Communications* 9, no. 1 (2018), doi:10.1038/s41467-017-02683-x.

14. Evanna L. Mills et al., "Itaconate is an anti-inflammatory metabolite that activates Nrf2 via alkylation of KEAP1," *Nature* (2018), doi:10.1038/ nature25986.

15. S. Reuter et al., "Oxidative stress, inflammation, and cancer: How are they linked?" *Free Radical Biology and Medicine* 49, no. 11 (2010): 1603–16, doi:10.1016/j.freeradbiomed.2010.09.006.

16. H. Kwon and J. E. Pessin, "Adipokines Mediate Inflammation and Insulin Resistance," *Frontiers in Endocrinology* 4 (2013): 71, doi:10.3389/fendo .2013.00071.

17. Anette Christ et al., "Western Diet Triggers NLRP3-Dependent Innate Immune Reprogramming," *Cell* 172, no. 1–2 (2018): 162.

18. Floris Fransen et al., "Aged Gut Microbiota Contributes to Systemical Inflammaging after Transfer to Germ-Free Mice," *Frontiers in Immunology* 8 (2017).
19. Bing Han et al., "Microbial Genetic Composition Tunes Host Longevity," *Cell* 169, no. 7 (2017): 1249.
20. S. V. Joseph et al., "Berries: anti-inflammatory effects in humans," *Journal of Agricultural and Food Chemistry* 62, no. 18 (May 2014): 3886–903, doi:10.1021/jf4044056.

    J. Goletzke et al., "Increased intake of carbohydrates from sources with a higher glycemic index and lower consumption of whole grains during puberty are prospectively associated with higher IL-6 concentrations in younger adulthood among healthy individuals," *Journal of Nutrition* 144, no. 10 (October 2014): 1586–93, doi:10.3945/jn.114.193391.

    Z. Li et al., "Hass avocado modulates postprandial vascular reactivity and postprandial inflammatory responses to a hamburger meal in healthy volunteers," *Food & Function* 4, no. 3 (February 2013): 384–91, doi:10.1039/c2fo30226h.
21. A. Sureda et al., "Adherence to the Mediterranean Diet and Inflammatory Markers," *Nutrients* 10, no. 1 (January 2018): E62, doi:10.3390/nu10010062.
22. L. K. Forsythe, J. M. Wallace, and M. B. Livingstone, "Obesity and inflammation: the effects of weight loss," *Nutrition Research Reviews* 21, no. 2 (December 2008): 117–33.
23. T. Kadowaki and T. Yamauchi, "Adiponectin and adiponectin receptors," *Endocrine Reviews* 26, no. 3 (May 2005): 439–51.

    Y. Miyoshi et al., "Association of serum adiponectin levels with breast cancer risk," *Clinical Cancer Research* 9, no. 15 (November 2003): 5699–704.

    R. Shibata et al., "Adiponectin protects against myocardial ischemia-reperfusion injury through AMPK- and COX-2-dependent mechanisms," *Nature Medicine* (October 2005): 1096–103.

    Y. Kamada, "Hypoadiponectinemia accelerates hepatic tumor formation in a nonalcoholic steatohepatitis mouse model," *Journal of Hepatology* 47, no. 4 (October 2007): 556–64.
24. W. S. Rosanna et al., "Lutein exerts anti-inflammatory effects in patients with coronary artery disease," *Atherosclerosis* 262 (2017): 87, doi:10.1016/j.atherosclerosis.2017.05.008.
25. S. Volpato, "Relationship of alcohol intake with inflammatory markers and plasminogen activator inhibitor-1 in well-functioning older adults: the Health, Aging, and Body Composition study," *Circulation* 109, no. 5 (February 2004): 607–12.
26. Iben Lundgaard et al., "Beneficial effects of low alcohol exposure, but adverse effects of high alcohol intake on glymphatic function," *Scientific Reports* 8, no. 1 (2018): doi:10.1038/s41598-018-20424-y.

27. H. J. Wang, S. Zakhari, and M. K. Jung, "Alcohol, inflammation, and gut-liver-brain interactions in tissue damage and disease development," *World Journal of Gastroenterology* 16, no. 11 (2010): 1304–1313.

28. M. S. Ellulu et al., "Effect of long chain omega-3 polyunsaturated fatty acids on inflammation and metabolic markers in hypertensive and/or diabetic obese adults: a randomized controlled trial," *Food & Nutrition Research* 60 (January 2016): 29268, doi:10.3402/fnr.v60.29268.

29. M. S. Ellulu et al., "Effect of vitamin C on inflammation and metabolic markers in hypertensive and/or diabetic obese adults: a randomized controlled trial," *Drug Design, Development and Therapy* 9 (2015): 3405–3412, doi:10.2147/DDDT.S83144.

Q. Jiang, "Natural forms of vitamin E: metabolism, antioxidant and anti-inflammatory activities and the role in disease prevention and therapy," *Free Radical Biology & Medicine* 72 (2014): 76–90, doi:10.1016/j.freeradbiomed.2014.03.035.

A. Tatar, "Anti-inflammatory and anti-oxidative effects of alpha-lipoic acid in experimentally induced acute otitis media," *Journal of Laryngology & Otology* 130, no. 7 (July 2016): 616–23, doi: 10.1017/S0022215116001183.

30. Y. Li, et al., "Quercetin, Inflammation and Immunity," *Nutrients* 8, no. 3 (2016): 167, doi:10.3390/nu8030167.

31. E. H. Lee, "A randomized study to establish the effects of spirulina in type 2 diabetes mellitus patients," *Nutrition Research and Practice* 2, no. 4 (Winter 2008): 295–300, doi:10.4162/nrp.2008.2.4.295.

32. Anne-Sophie Wedell-Neergaard, "Low fitness is associated with abdominal adiposity and low-grade inflammation independent of BMI," *PLoS ONE* 13, no. 1 (2018): e0190645, doi:10.1371/journal.pone.0190645.

33. L. K. Forsythe and J. M. Wallace, "Obesity and inflammation: the effects of weight loss," *Nutrition Research Review* 21, no. 2 (December 2008): 117–33.

34. P. Muñoz-Cánoves, "Interleukin-6 myokine signaling in skeletal muscle: a double-edged sword?" *FEBS Journal* 280, no. 17 (September 2013): 4131–48.

35. R. A. B. Nunes et al., "High-sensitivity C–reactive protein levels and treadmill exercise test responses in men and women without overt heart disease," *Experimental & Clinical Cardiology* 18, no. 2 (2013): 124–128.

36. S. Dimitrov, E. Hulteng, and S. Hong, "Inflammation and exercise: Inhibition of monocytic intracellular TNF production by acute exercise via β2-adrenergic activation," *Brain, Behavior, and Immunity* 61 (March 2017): 60–68.

37. S. Gill et al., "The Impact of a 24-h Ultra-Marathon on Circulatory Endotoxin and Cytokine Profile," *International Journal of Sports Medicine* (2015), doi:10.1055/s-0034-1398535.

38. F. Z. Madani et al., "Hemostatic, inflammatory, and oxidative markers in pesticide user farmers," *Biomarkers* 21, no. 2 (2016): 138–45, doi:10.3109/13 54750X.2015.1118545.

P. Y. Bai, "The association between total phthalate concentration and non-communicable diseases and chronic inflammation in South Australian urban dwelling men," *Environmental Research* 158 (October 2017): 366–372, doi:10.1016/j.envres.2017.06.021.

Y. J. Choi, K. H. Ha, and D. J. Kim, "Exposure to bisphenol A is directly associated with inflammation in healthy Korean adults," *Environmental Science and Pollution Research* 24, no. 1 (January 2017): 284–290.

A. Y. Leem et al., "Relationship between blood levels of heavy metals and lung function based on the Korean National Health and Nutrition Examination Survey IV–V," *International Journal of Chronic Obstructive Pulmonary Disease* 10 (2015): 1559–1570, doi:10.2147/COPD.S86182.

39. B. B. Gump et al., "Fish Consumption, Low-Level Mercury, Lipids, and Inflammatory Markers in Children," *Environmental Research* 112 (2012): 204–211, doi:10.1016/j.envres.2011.10.002.

40. P. Dadvand et al., "Air pollution and biomarkers of systemic inflammation and tissue repair in COPD patients," *European Respiratory Journal* 44, no. 3 (2014): 603–13, doi:10.1183/09031936.00168813.

41. P. L. Minciullo et al., "Cytokine Network Involvement in Subjects Exposed to Benzene," *Journal of Immunology Research* (2014): 937987, doi:10.1155/2014/937987.

42. J. Yang et al., "Importance of indoor dust biological ultrafine particles in the pathogenesis of chronic inflammatory lung diseases," *Environmental Health and Toxicology* 32 (2017): e2017021, doi:10.5620/eht.e2017021.

43. L. F. Lima et al., "Short-term exposure to formaldehyde promotes oxidative damage and inflammation in the trachea and diaphragm muscle of adult rats," *Annals of Anatomy* 202 (November 2015): 45–51, doi:10.1016/j.aanat.2015.08.003.

44. M. R. Irwin, R. Olmstead, and J. E. Carroll, "Sleep Disturbance, Sleep Duration, and Inflammation: A Systematic Review and Meta-Analysis of Cohort Studies and Experimental Sleep Deprivation," *Biological Psychiatry* 80, no. 1 (July 2016): 40–52, doi:10.1016/j.biopsych.2015.05.014.

45. Elsevier, "Loss Of Sleep, Even For A Single Night, Increases Inflammation In The Body," *ScienceDaily* 4 (September 2008), https://www.sciencedaily.com/releases/2008/09/080902075211.htm.

46. M. R. Irwin, R. Olmstead, and J. E. Carroll, "Sleep Disturbance, Sleep Duration, and Inflammation: A Systematic Review and Meta-Analysis of Cohort Studies and Experimental Sleep Deprivation," *Biological Psychiatry* 80, no. 1 (July 2016): 40–52, doi:10.1016/j.biopsych.2015.05.014.

47. Stephanie J. Wilson et al., "Shortened sleep fuels inflammatory responses to marital conflict: Emotion regulation matters," *Psychoneuroendocrinology* 79: 74–83, doi:10.1016/j.psyneuen.2017.02.015.

Chapter 8.   The Fifth Key: Managing Metabolism

1. Christopher R. Martens et al., "Chronic nicotinamide riboside supplementation is well-tolerated and elevates NAD in healthy middle-aged and older adults," *Nature Communications* (2018).
2. L. Fontana, L. Partridge, and V. D. Longo, "Extending healthy life span— from yeast to humans," *Science* 328 (2010): 321–26.
3. N. Barzilai et al., "The critical role of metabolic pathways in aging," *Diabetes* 61, no. 6 (2012): 1315–22.
4. J. Kim et al., "AMPK and mTOR regulate autophagy through direct phosphorylation of Ulk1," *Nature Cell Biology* 13, no. 2 (2011): 132–41.
5. A. Martin-Montalvo and R. de Cabo, "Mitochondrial metabolic reprogramming induced by calorie restriction," *Antioxidant and Redox Signaling* 19, no. 3 (July 2013): 310–20, doi:10.1089/ars.2012.4866.

     P. J. Fernandez-Marcos and J. Auwerx, "Regulation of PGC-1α, a nodal regulator of mitochondrial biogenesis," *The American Journal of Clinical Nutrition* 93, no. 4 (2011): 884S–890S, doi:10.3945/ajcn.110.001917.

     R. Tao et al., "Sirt3-mediated deacetylation of evolutionarily conserved lysine 122 regulates MnSOD activity in response to stress," *Molecular Cell* 40 (2010): 893–904.
6. B. Schumacher et al, "Delayed and accelerated aging share common longevity assurance mechanisms," *PLoS Genetics* 4 (2008): e1000161.
7. J. A. Mattison et al., "Impact of caloric restriction on health and survival in rhesus monkeys from the NIA study," *Nature* 489, no. 7415 (2012): 318–321.
8. Leanne M. Redman et al., "Metabolic Slowing and Reduced Oxidative Damage with Sustained Caloric Restriction Support the Rate of Living and Oxidative Damage Theories of Aging," *Cell Metabolism* (2018), doi:10.1016/j.cmet.2018.02.019.
9. V. N. Anisimov et al., "If started early in life, metformin treatment increases life span and postpones tumors in female SHR mice," *Aging* 3 (2011): 148–157.
10. S. C. Chao, "Induction of sirtuin-1 signaling by resveratrol induces human chondrosarcoma cell apoptosis and exhibits antitumor activity," *Scientific Reports* 7, no. 1 (June 2017): 3180, doi:10.1038/s41598-017-03635-7.
11. Sonia Navarro et al., "Inhaled resveratrol treatments slow aging-related degenerative changes in mouse lung," *Thorax* (2017), doi:thoraxjnl-2016 -208964.
12. D. E. Harrison et al., "Rapamycin fed late in life extends lifespan in genetically heterogeneous mice," *Nature* 460 (2009): 392–395.
13. S. C. Johnson, P. S. Rabinovitch, and M. Kaeberlein, "mTOR is a key modulator of ageing and age-related disease," *Nature* 493, no. 7432 (2013): 338–345, doi:10.1038/nature11861.
14. E. Kraig et al., "A randomized control trial to establish the feasibility and

safety of rapamycin treatment in an older human cohort: Immunological, physical performance, and cognitive effects," *Experimental Gerontology* 105 (May 2018): 53–69, doi:10.1016/j.exger.2017.12.026.

15. B. K. Kennedy and D. W. Lamming, "The Mechanistic Target of Rapamycin: The Grand ConducTOR of Metabolism and Aging," *Cell Metabolism* 23, no. 6 (June 2016): 990–1003, doi:10.1016/j.cmet.2016.05.009.

16. Abhirup Das et al., "Impairment of an Endothelial NAD^+-H_2S Signaling Network Is a Reversible Cause of Vascular Aging," *Cell* 173, no.1 (2018): 74, doi:10.1016/j.cell.2018.02.008.

17. G. A. Bell et al., "Use of glucosamine and chondroitin in relation to mortality," *European Journal of Epidemiology* 27, no. 8 (August 2012): 593–603, doi:10.1007/s10654-012-9714-6.

18. Sandra Weimer et al., "D-Glucosamine supplementation extends life span of nematodes and of ageing mice," *Nature Communications* 5 (2014): doi:10.1038/ncomms4563.

19. F. He et al., "Serum Polychlorinated Biphenyls Increase and Oxidative Stress Decreases with a Protein-Pacing Caloric Restriction Diet in Obese Men and Women," *International Journal of Environmental Research and Public Health* 14, no. 1 (January 2017), pii:E59, doi:10.3390/ijerph1401 0059.

20. T. Moro et al., "Effects of eight weeks of time-restricted feeding (16/8) on basal metabolism, maximal strength, body composition, inflammation, and cardiovascular risk factors in resistance-trained males," *Journal of Translational Medicine* 14, no.1 (2016): 290.

21. Bodo C. Melnik, Swen Malte John, and Gerd Schmitz, "Over-stimulation of insulin/IGF-1 signaling by Western diet may promote diseases of civilization," *Nutrition & Metabolism* (2011) 8:41 doi.org/10.1186/1743-7075-8-41.

22. K. Tsubota, "The first human clinical study for NMN has started in Japan," *NPJ Aging and Mechanisms of Disease* 2 (2016): 16021, doi:10.1038/npjamd .2016.21.

23. Kathryn F. Mills et al., "Long-Term Administration of Nicotinamide Mononucleotide Mitigates Age-Associated Physiological Decline in Mice," *Cell Metabolism* (October 2016): doi:10.1016/j.cmet.2016.09.013.

24. A. Combes et al., "Exercise-induced metabolic fluctuations influence AMPK, p38-MAPK and CaMKII phosphorylation in human skeletal muscle," *Physiological Reports* 3, no. 9 (2015): e12462, doi:10.14814/phy2 .12462.

25. C. C. Huang et al., "Effect of Exercise Training on Skeletal Muscle SIRT1 and PGC-1α Expression Levels in Rats of Different Age," *International Journal of Medical Sciences* 13, no.4 (2016): 260–70, doi:10.7150/ijms.14586.

26. B. J. Gurd et al., "High-intensity interval training increases SIRT1 activity in human skeletal muscle," *Applied Physiology, Nutrition, and Metabolism* 35, no. 3 (June 2010): 350–7.

27. T. Groennebaek and K. Vissing, "Impact of Resistance Training on Skeletal Muscle Mitochondrial Biogenesis, Content, and Function," *Frontiers in Physiology* 8 (2017): 713, doi:10.3389/fphys.2017.00713.

28. R. Kakigi et al., "Whey protein intake after resistance exercise activates mTOR signaling in a dose-dependent manner in human skeletal muscle," *European Journal of Applied Physiology* 144, no. 4 (April 2014): 735–42, doi:10.1007/s00421-013-2812-7.

29. J. Zhang et al., "Extended Wakefulness: Compromised Metabolics in and Degeneration of Locus Ceruleus Neurons," *Journal of Neuroscience* 34, no. 12 (2014): 4418, doi:10.1523/JNEUROSCI.5025-12.2014.

Chapter 9. The Sixth Key: Tackling Telomeres

1. Colter Mitchell et al., "Father Loss and Child Telomere Length. Pediatrics," (2017): e20163245, doi:10.1542/peds.2016-3245.

2. A. Z. Pollack, K. Rivers, and K. A. Ahrens, "Parity associated with telomere length among US reproductive age women," *Human Reproduction* (February 2018), doi:10.1093/humrep/dey024.

3. C. K. Barha et al., "Number of Children and Telomere Length in Women: A Prospective, Longitudinal Evaluation, S. Helle ed., *PLoS ONE* 11, no. 1 (2016): e0146424, doi:10.1371/journal.pone.0146424.

4. D. W. Bianchi et al., "Male fetal progenitor cells persist in maternal blood for as long as 27 years postpartum," *Proceedings of the National Academy of Sciences of the United States of America* 93 (1996): 705–8.

5. T. Z. Nazari-Shafti and J. P. Cooke, "Telomerase Therapy to Reverse Cardiovascular Senescence," *Methodist DeBakey Cardiovascular Journal* 11, no. 3 (2015): 172–175, doi:10.14797/mdcj-11-3-172.

6. Elisa Varela et al., "Generation of mice with longer and better preserved telomeres in the absence of genetic manipulations," *Nature Communications* 7 (2016): 11739, doi:10.1038/ncomms11739.

7. Shengda Lin et al., "Distributed hepatocytes expressing telomerase repopulate the liver in homeostasis and injury," *Nature* (2018): doi:10.1038/s41586-018-0004-7.

8. J. Choi, S. R. Fauce, and R. B. Effros, "Reduced telomerase activity in human T lymphocytes exposed to cortisol," *Brain Behavior and Immunity* 22 (May 2008): 600–05.

9. D. Jurk et al., "Chronic inflammation induces telomere dysfunction and accelerates ageing in mice," *Nature Communications* 2 (June 2014): 4172.

10. D. Ornish et al., "Effect of comprehensive lifestyle changes on telomerase activity and telomere length in men with biopsy-proven low-risk prostate cancer: 5-year follow-up of a descriptive pilot study," *The Lancet Oncology* (2013).

11. Shiqin Xiong et al., "PGC-1α Modulates Telomere Function and DNA Damage in Protecting against Aging-Related Chronic Diseases," *Cell Reports* (2015).

12. K. B. Min and J. Y. Min, "Association between leukocyte telomere length and serum carotenoid in US adults," *European Journal of Nutrition* 56, no. 3 (April 2017): 1045–52, doi:10.1007/s00394-016-1152-x.

13. A. Barden et al., "n-3 Fatty Acid Supplementation and Leukocyte Telomere Length in Patients with Chronic Kidney Disease," *Nutrients* 8, no. 3 (2016): 175, doi:10.3390/nu8030175.

14. Janice K. Kiecolt-Glaser et al., "Omega-3 supplementation lowers inflammation in healthy middle-aged and older adults: A randomized controlled trial," *Brain, Behavior, and Immunity* 26, no. 6 (2012): 988, doi:10.1016/j.bbi.2012.05.011.

15. C. W. Leung et al., "Soda and cell aging: associations between sugar-sweetened beverage consumption and leukocyte telomere length in healthy adults from the National Health and Nutrition Examination Surveys," *American Journal of Public Health* 104, no. 12 (December 2014): 2425–31, doi:10.2105/AJPH.2014.302151.

16. A. M. Fretts et al., "Processed Meat, but Not Unprocessed Red Meat, Is Inversely Associated with Leukocyte Telomere Length in the Strong Heart Family Study," *The Journal of Nutrition* 146, no. 10 (2016): 2013–18, doi:10.3945/jn.116.234922.

17. L. A. Tucker, "Caffeine consumption and telomere length in men and women of the National Health and Nutrition Examination Survey (NHANES)," *Nutrition and Metabolism* 14 (January 2017): 10, doi:10.1186/s12986-017-0162-x.

18. L. Latifovic et al., "The Influence of Alcohol Consumption, Cigarette Smoking, and Physical Activity on Leukocyte Telomere Length," *Cancer Epidemiology, Biomarkers & Prevention* 25, no. 2 (February 2016): 374–80, doi:10.1158/1055-9965.EPI-14-1364.

19. Larry A. Tucker, "Physical activity and telomere length in U.S. men and women: An NHANES investigation," *Preventive Medicine* 100 (2017): 145.

20. European Society of Cardiology, "Weight loss from bariatric surgery appears to reverse premature aging: Patients had longer telomeres and less inflammation two years later," *ScienceDaily* (July 2016).

21. Per Sjögren et al., "Stand up for health—avoiding sedentary behaviour might lengthen your telomeres: secondary outcomes from a physical activity RCT in older people," *British Journal of Sports Medicine* (September 2014): doi:10.1136/bjsports-2013-093342.

22. Aladdin H. Shadyab et al., "Associations of Accelerometer-Measured and Self-Reported Sedentary Time With Leukocyte Telomere Length in Older Women," *American Journal of Epidemiology* (January 2017): doi:10.1093/aje/kww196.

23. H. Lavretsky et al., "A pilot study of yogic meditation for family dementia caregivers with depressive symptoms: Effects on mental health, cognition, and telomerase activity," *International Journal of Geriatric Psychiatry* 28, no. 1 (2013): 57–65, doi:10.1002/gps.3790.

24. M. Collins et al., "Athletes with exercise-associated fatigue have abnormally short muscle DNA telomeres," *Medicine and Science in Sports and Exercise* 35, no. 9 (September 2003): 1524–8.

25. A. T. Ludlow et al., "Relationship between physical activity level, telomere length, and telomerase activity," *Medicine and Science in Sports and Exercise* 40, no. 10 (2008): 1764–71.

26. M. J. Laye et al., "Increased shelterin mRNA expression in peripheral blood mononuclear cells and skeletal muscle following an ultra-long-distance running event," *Journal of Applied Physiology* 112, no. 5 (2012): 773–81.

27. I. B. Ø. Østhus et al., "Telomere Length and Long-Term Endurance Exercise: Does Exercise Training Affect Biological Age? A Pilot Study," ed. A. Lucia, *PLoS One* 7, no. 12 (2012): e52769, doi:10.1371/journal.pone .0052769.

28. M. B. Mathur et al., "Perceived Stress and Telomere Length: A Systematic Review, Meta-Analysis, and Methodologic Considerations for Advancing the Field," *Brain, Behavior, and Immunity* 54 (2016): 158–169, doi:10.1016/ j.bbi.2016.02.002.

29. Yiqiang Zhan et al., "Telomere Length Shortening and Alzheimer Disease—A Mendelian Randomization Study," *JAMA Neurology* 72, no. 10 (2015): 1202–1203.

30. Brigham and Women's Hospital, "Anxiety linked to shortened telomeres, accelerated aging," *ScienceDaily* (July 2012): Retrieved March 20, 2018 from https://www.sciencedaily.com/releases/2012/07/120711210102.htm.

31. Denise Aydinonat et al., "Social Isolation Shortens Telomeres in African Grey Parrots (*Psittacus erithacus erithacus*)," *PLoS One* 9, no. 4 (2014): e93839, doi:10.1371/journal.pone.0093839.

32. Mijung Park et al., "Where You Live May Make You Old: The Association between Perceived Poor Neighborhood Quality and Leukocyte Telomere Length," *PLOS One* 10, no. 6 (2015): e0128460, doi:10.1371/journal. pone.0128460.

33. T. Cabeza de Baca et al., "Sexual intimacy in couples is associated with longer telomere length," *Psychoneuroendocrinology* 81 (July 2017): 46–51, doi:10.1016/j.psyneuen.2017.03.022.

34. M. Jackowska et al., "Short sleep duration is associated with shorter telomere length in healthy men: findings from the Whitehall II cohort study," *PLoS One* 7, no. 10 (2012): e47292, doi:10.1371/journal.pone .0047292.

35. J. Huzen et al., "Telomere length loss due to smoking and metabolic traits," *Journal of Internal Medicine* 275 (2014): 155–63.

36. Eunice Y. Lee et al., "Traffic-Related Air Pollution and Telomere Length in Children and Adolescents Living in Fresno, CA," *Journal of Occupational and Environmental Medicine* 59, no. 5 (2017): 446, doi:10.1097/JOM.000 0000000000996.

37. Frederica Perera et al., "Shorter telomere length in cord blood associated with prenatal air pollution exposure: Benefits of intervention," *Environment International* (2018), doi:10.1016/j.envint.2018.01.005.
38. S. Ribero et al., "Acne and telomere length. A new spectrum between senescence and apoptosis pathways," *Journal of Investigative Dermatology* (2016).

Chapter 10. Before We Begin

1. A. Z. Pollock, K. Rivers, and K. A. Ahrean, "Parity associated with telomere length among US reproductive age women," *Human Reproduction* (February 2018), doi:10.1093/humrep/dey024.
2. C. K. Barha et al., "Number of Children and Telomere Length in Women: A Prospective, Longitudinal Evaluation," ed. S. Helle, *PLoS ONE* 11, no. 1 (2016): e0146424, doi:10.1371/journal.pone.0146424.

Chapter 11. The 6 Keys Lifestyle Strategy

1. M. S. Ball and B. Vernon, "A review on how meditation could be used to comfort the terminally ill," *Palliative Support & Care* 13, no. 5 (October 2015): 1469–72, doi:10.1017/S1478951514001308.

    A. J. Lang et al., "The theoretical and empirical basis for meditation as an intervention for PTSD," *Behavior Modification* 36, no. 6 (November 2012): 759–86, doi:10.1177/0145445512441200.

    M. Speca et al., "A randomized, wait-list controlled clinical trial: the effect of a mindfulness meditation-based stress reduction program on mood and symptoms of stress in cancer outpatients," *Psychosomatic Medicine* 62, no. 5 (September–October 2000): 613–22.

    E. H. Kozasa et al., "The effects of meditation-based interventions on the treatment of fibromyalgia," *Current Pain and Headache Reports* 15, no. 5 (October 2012): 383–7, doi:10.1007/s11916-012-0285-8.
2. E. R. Kasala et al., "Effect of meditation on neurophysiological changes in stress mediated depression," *Complementary Therapies in Clinical Practice* 20, no. 1 (February 2014): 74–80, doi: 10.1016/j.ctcp.2013.10.001.
3. J. D. Creswell et al., "Mindfulness-Based Stress Reduction training reduces loneliness and pro-inflammatory gene expression in older adults: a small randomized controlled trial," *Brain, Behavior, and Immunity* 26, no. 7 (October 2012): 1095–101.

Chapter 12. The 6 Keys Mind-Body Strategy

1. B. R. Levy et al., "Positive age beliefs protect against dementia even among elders with high-risk gene," ed. S. D. Ginsberg, *PLoS ONE* 13, no. 2 (2018): e0191004, doi:10.1371/journal.pone.0191004.
2. P. L. Hill and N. A. Turiano, "Purpose in life as a predictor of mortality across adulthood," *Psychological Science* 25, no. 7 (July 2014): 1482–6.

Index

About the Authors

Jillian Michaels is the most prominent health and fitness expert in the world. She has dominated the health and wellness space with eight *New York Times*–bestselling books; hit television shows; immensely successful workout DVDs; her My Fitness diet and exercise app, which was voted best of 2017 by both Apple and Google; and her award-winning podcast. Through her platforms, she has built an international community of followers 100 million–plus strong. Jillian's Empowered Media is dedicated to providing total-life solutions for all aspects of living well, including fitness, nutrition, self-help, and overall lifestyle. She has a fierce passion for learning and is an avid world traveler. She is the mother of two.

Myatt Murphy is a journalist who has written for many of the world's top publications, including *Better Homes & Gardens, Men's Health, AARP,* and *Cooking Light.* He is the author of many bestselling books and has also written books with many of today's top lifestyle specialists, including Harley Pasternak, Gunnar Peterson, and Jenna Wolfe.